T0249746

Diabetes in Older Adults

Editor

S. SETHU K. REDDY

CLINICS IN GERIATRIC MEDICINE

www.geriatric.theclinics.com

August 2020 • Volume 36 • Number 3

ELSEVIER

1600 John F. Kennedy Boulevard • Suite 1800 • Philadelphia, Pennsylvania, 19103-2899

http://www.theclinics.com

CLINICS IN GERIATRIC MEDICINE Volume 36, Number 3
August 2020 ISSN 0749–0690, ISBN-13: 978-0-323-76062-1

Editor: Katerina Heidhausen
Developmental Editor: Laura Fisher

© 2020 Elsevier Inc. All rights reserved.

This periodical and the individual contributions contained in it are protected under copyright by Elsevier, and the following terms and conditions apply to their use:

Photocopying
Single photocopies of single articles may be made for personal use as allowed by national copyright laws. Permission of the Publisher and payment of a fee is required for all other photocopying, including multiple or systematic copying, copying for advertising or promotional purposes, resale, and all forms of document delivery. Special rates are available for educational institutions that wish to make photocopies for non-profit educational classroom use. For information on how to seek permission visit www.elsevier.com/permissions or call: (+44) 1865 843830 (UK)/(+1) 215 239 3804 (USA).

Derivative Works
Subscribers may reproduce tables of contents or prepare lists of articles including abstracts for internal circulation within their institutions. Permission of the Publisher is required for resale or distribution outside the institution. Permission of the Publisher is required for all other derivative works, including compilations and translations (please consult www.elsevier.com/permissions).

Electronic Storage or Usage
Permission of the Publisher is required to store or use electronically any material contained in this periodical, including any article or part of an article (please consult www.elsevier.com/permissions). Except as outlined above, no part of this publication may be reproduced, stored in a retrieval system or transmitted in any form or by any means, electronic, mechanical, photocopying, recording or otherwise, without prior written permission of the Publisher.

Notice
No responsibility is assumed by the Publisher for any injury and/or damage to persons or property as a matter of products liability, negligence or otherwise, or from any use or operation of any methods, products, instructions or ideas contained in the material herein. Because of rapid advances in the medical sciences, in particular, independent verification of diagnoses and drug dosages should be made.

Although all advertising material is expected to conform to ethical (medical) standards, inclusion in this publication does not constitute a guarantee or endorsement of the quality or value of such product or of the claims made of it by its manufacturer.

Clinics in Geriatric Medicine (ISSN 0749-0690) is published quarterly by Elsevier Inc., 360 Park Avenue South, New York, NY 10010-1710. Months of issue are February, May, August, and November. Business and Editorial Offices: 1600 John F. Kennedy Blvd., Suite 1800, Philadelphia, PA 191023-2899. Periodicals postage paid at New York, NY, and additional mailing offices. Subscription prices are $289.00 per year (US individuals), $664.00 per year (US institutions), $100.00 per year (US & Canadian student/resident), $320.00 per year (Canadian individuals), $841.00 per year (Canadian institutions), $414.00 per year (international individuals), $841.00 per year (international institutions), and $195.00 per year (international student/resident). Foreign air speed delivery is included in all *Clinics* subscription prices. All prices are subject to change without notice. POSTMASTER: Send address changes to *Clinics in Geriatric Medicine,* Elsevier Health Sciences Division, Subscription Customer Service, 3251 Riverport Lane, Maryland Heights, MO 63043. **Telephone: 1-800-654-2452 (U.S. and Canada); 314-447-8871 (outside U.S. and Canada). Fax: 314-447-8029. E-mail:** journalscustomerservice-usa@elsevier.com **(for print support)** or journalsonlinesupport-usa@elsevier.com **(for online support).**

Reprints. For copies of 100 or more, of articles in this publication, please contact the Commercial Reprints Department, Elsevier Inc., 360 Park Avenue South, New York, New York 10010-1710. Tel.: 212-633-3874; Fax: 212-633-3820, E-mail: reprints@elsevier.com.

Clinics in Geriatric Medicine is covered in *MEDLINE/PubMed (Index Medicus), EMBASE/Excerpta Medica, Current Contents/Clinical Medicine (CC/CM),* and the *Cumulative Index to Nursing & Allied Health Literature.*

Contributors

EDITOR

S. SETHU K. REDDY, MD, MBA
Professor and Chair of Medicine, Professor, Department of Internal Medicine, Central Michigan University College of Medicine, Mount Pleasant, Michigan, USA

AUTHORS

AHMED ABDELHAFIZ, MD, FRCP
Department of Geriatric Medicine, Rotherham General Hospital, Rotherham, United Kingdom

CHARLES M. ALEXANDER, MD
Alexander Associates LLC, Gwynedd Valley, Pennsylvania, USA

RAWAN AMIR, MBBS
Internal Medicine Resident, Central Michigan University, Saginaw, Michigan, USA

SANJEEB BHATTACHARYA, MD, FACC
Section of Heart Failure and Cardiac Transplant Medicine, Cleveland Clinic, Cleveland, Ohio, USA

GEORGIA M. DAVIS, MD
Assistant Professor, Department of Medicine, Division of Endocrinology, Emory University School of Medicine, Atlanta, Georgia, USA

KRISTEN DeCARLO, MD
Endocrinology Fellow, Division of Endocrinology, Metabolism and Molecular Medicine, Northwestern University Feinberg School of Medicine, Chicago, Illinois, USA

JERRY ESTEP, MD, FACC, FASE
Section Head, Section of Heart Failure and Cardiac Transplant Medicine, Cleveland Clinic, Cleveland, Ohio, USA

CHARLES FAIMAN, MD, FRCPC, MACE
Retired, Head, Department of Endocrinology, Cleveland Clinic, Cleveland, Ohio, USA

ARDESHIR HASHMI, MD, FACP
Center for Geriatric Medicine, Endowed Chair for Geriatric Innovation, Cleveland Clinic Center for Geriatric Medicine, Cleveland, Ohio, USA

BYRON J. HOOGWERF, MD, FACP, FACE
Retired Staff, Diabetes, Endocrinology and Metabolism, Cleveland Clinic, Cleveland, Ohio, USA; Clinical Professor, Central Michigan University, College of Medicine, Mount Pleasant, Michigan, USA

MARK PAUL MacEACHERN, MLIS
Informationist, Taubman Health Sciences Library, University of Michigan, Ann Arbor, Michigan, USA

ALESSANDRO MANTOVANI, MD
Section of Endocrinology, Diabetes, and Metabolism, University and Azienda Ospedaliera Universitaria Integrata of Verona, Verona, Italy

ADI MEHTA, MD, FRCPC, FACE
Endocrinology and Metabolism Institute, Cleveland Clinic, Cleveland, Ohio, USA

FRANCISCO J. PASQUEL, MD, MPH
Assistant Professor, Department of Medicine, Division of Endocrinology, Emory University School of Medicine, Assistant Professor of Medicine, Emory University, Atlanta, Georgia, USA

SATHYA REDDY, MD
Staff Physician, Cleveland Clinic, Lorain, Ohio, USA

S. SETHU K. REDDY, MD, MBA
Professor and Chair of Medicine, Professor, Department of Internal Medicine, Central Michigan University College of Medicine, Mount Pleasant, Michigan, USA

ALAN SINCLAIR, MSc, MD, FRCP
Foundation for Diabetes Research in Older People, Diabetes Frail Ltd, Droitwich Spa, United Kingdom; Kings College, London, United Kingdom

RAM D. SRIRAM, PhD
National Institute of Standards and Technology

SARA SUHL, BS
Research Associate, dQ&A Diabetes Research, San Francisco, California, USA

KHINE SWE, MD,
Resident Physician, St. Mary's Ascension, Central Michigan University College of Medicine, Saginaw, Michigan, USA

MENGHEE TAN, MD
Professor Emeritus, Division of Metabolism, Endocrinology and Diabetes, Department of Internal Medicine, University of Michigan, Ann Arbor, Michigan, USA

GIOVANNI TARGHER, MD
Section of Endocrinology, Diabetes, and Metabolism, University and Azienda Ospedaliera Universitaria Integrata of Verona, Verona, Italy

ZEHRA TEKIN, MD
Clinical Fellow, Endocrinology, Diabetes and Metabolism Institute, Cleveland Clinic Foundation, Cleveland, Ohio, USA

GUILLERMO E. UMPIERREZ, MD, CDE
Professor, Department of Medicine, Division of Endocrinology, Emory University School of Medicine, Atlanta, Georgia, USA

AMISHA WALLIA, MD, MS
Assistant Professor, Division of Endocrinology, Metabolism and Molecular Medicine, Northwestern University Feinberg School of Medicine, Chicago, Illinois, USA

ROBERT S. ZIMMERMAN, MD, FACE
Clinical Assistant Professor of Medicine, Vice Chairman, Director of Diabetes Center, Endocrinology, Diabetes and Metabolism Institute, Cleveland Clinic Foundation, Cleveland, Ohio, USA

GIACOMO ZOPPINI, MD, PhD
Section of Endocrinology, Diabetes, and Metabolism, University and Azienda Ospedaliera Universitaria Integrata of Verona, Verona, Italy

Contents

on patients' self-care tasks. With further progression of dementia and the development of behavioral problems, the challenge to carers and health care professionals looking after these patients is significant. Therefore, clinical trials are needed to explore the impact of novel hypoglycemic therapy on cognitive function as an important outcome in this population.

People with diabetes mellitus (DM), especially those who are older, are at higher risk for premature morbidity and mortality related to atherosclerotic cardiovascular disease (ASCVD). Clinical practice guidelines recommend statin therapy for people with DM ages 40 to 75 years. The evidence for those greater than 75 years of age is relatively limited at present. Other health problems should be considered when planning ASCVD primary prevention in adults ages greater than 75 years with DM. Clinicians should discuss the risks and benefits of each plan with these patients and their caregivers.

International Diabetes Federation estimates that there are more than a half-billion adults ages 20 to 79 years worldwide who have diabetes mellitus (DM) and that the global health care expenditure for adults with DM in 2015 was $673 billion. Nonadherence and nonpersistence to prescribed type 2 DM medications are common and remain a barrier to optimal health outcomes. There is a high prevalence of nonadherence among older adults. Research has focused on prevalence and predictors of adherence, research methodologies, and development of measures of adherence. Improvements hopefully will result in better disease monitoring, medication adherence, and reduced rates of diabetes complications.

Diabetes is one of the world's fastest growing health challenges. Insulin therapy remains a useful regimen for many elderly patients, such as those with moderate to severe hyperglycemia, type 1 diabetes, hyperglycemic emergencies, and those who fail to maintain glucose control on non-insulin agents alone. Recent clinical trials have shown that several non-insulin agents as monotherapy, or in combination with low doses of basal insulin, have comparable efficacy and potential safety advantages to complex insulin therapy regimens. Determining the most appropriate diabetes management plan for older hospitalized patients requires consideration of many factors to prevent poor outcomes related to dysglycemia.

Diabetes mellitus has become a global threat, especially in the emerging economies. In the United States, there are about 24 million people with diabetes mellitus. Diabetes represents a trove of physiologic and sociologic data that are only superficially understood by the health care system. Artificial intelligence can address many problems posed by the prevalence of diabetes mellitus and the impact of diabetes on individual and societal health. We provide a brief overview of artificial intelligence and discuss

Nonalcoholic fatty liver disease (NAFLD) is common in older patients with type 2 diabetes. In older patients with type 2 diabetes, the presence of NAFLD is associated with a higher risk of hepatic (eg, nonalcoholic steatohepatitis, cirrhosis, and hepatocellular carcinoma) and extrahepatic (eg, cardiovascular disease, sarcopenia, and dementia) complications than that observed in other patient groups. For this reason, appropriate identification and management of NAFLD are clinically relevant particularly in the group of older patients with type 2 diabetes. In this regard, clinicians should consider the peculiar characteristics of elderly patients, such as frailty, multimorbidity, and polypharmacy.

CLINICS IN GERIATRIC MEDICINE

FORTHCOMING ISSUES

November 2020
Healthy Aging
Susan M. Friedman, *Editor*

February 2021
Gastroenterology
Amir E. Soumekh and Philip O. Katz,
Editors

May 2021
Sleep in the Elderly
Steven H. Feinsilver and Margarita Oks,
Editors

RECENT ISSUES

May 2020
Geriatric Psychiatry
Dan G. Blazer and Susan K. Schultz,
Editors

February 2020
Parkinson Disease
Carlos Singer and Stephen Reich, *Editors*

November 2019
Cardiac Rehabilitation for Older Adults
Daniel E. Forman, *Editor*

SERIES OF RELATED INTEREST

Medical Clinics of North America
Primary Care: Clinics in Office Practice
Endocrinology & Metabolism Clinics

THE CLINICS ARE AVAILABLE ONLINE!
Access your subscription at:
www.theclinics.com

Preface

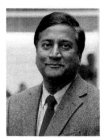

S. Sethu K. Reddy
Editor

The human world is facing an aging phenomenon; in 2015, 901 million people were aged ≥60 years, with most of these individuals living in developed countries. This number is expected to more than double by 2050, reaching 2.1 billion (ie, 20% of the global population). Moreover, the number of people aged >80 years is growing more rapidly than the general older adult population. Approximately 14% of the older adult population (125 million) were ≥80 years in 2015, and this will triple by 2050, reaching 434 million (approximately 20% of the senior population).[1] This phenomenon puts clear pressure on health care systems and social service support structures.

As our patients are living longer, we cannot afford to be ageist. We cannot ignore cardiorenal issues, and we must consider the utility of existing strategies to improve cardiac health and preserve renal function in older adults. In particular, congestive heart failure and diabetes are frequently comorbidities in older adults, and we are learning more about the interplay between the 2 syndromes. Optimal management of both conditions should lead to greater quality and quantity of life.

Prevention of diabetes and heart disease may involve more aggressive management of nonalcoholic hepatic steatosis or nonalcoholic fatty liver disease. We have known of the link for decades, but we appear to be on the cusp of medical interventions that, it is hoped, will alter the natural history of this common but often forgotten condition.

The medical tsunami before us includes the double scenario of cognitive decline and diabetes. As we become more successful in preventing heart disease, osteoporosis, and renal failure, our patients are getting older with more cognitive decline resulting in diabetes regimens more challenging to implement. Here too is a pathophysiologic 2-way street where hypoglycemia may beget cognitive decline and vice versa. In addition to the risk of hypoglycemia, we must also be familiar with the pros and cons of our existing therapeutic armamentarium in the changing physiology of an older adult.

Technology and increasing incorporation of artificial intelligence promise to be a great help. Preventing hypoglycemia, developing closed-loop systems, increasing adherence to medications, and ensuring patient safety will improve diabetes control and improve the lives of our patients and their loved ones. Every patient could have a "SmartCoach" or an "iCoach."

Clin Geriatr Med 36 (2020) xiii–xiv
https://doi.org/10.1016/j.cger.2020.05.001
0749-0690/20/© 2020 Published by Elsevier Inc.

geriatric.theclinics.com

I am grateful to phenomenal friends and colleagues who have contributed several hundred years of collective clinical experience to the contents that follows. I hope that you will find these illuminating as well as practical in your care of older adults with diabetes.

S. Sethu K. Reddy
CMU College of Medicine
CMED 2419
Mt. Pleasant, MI 48859, USA

E-mail address:
sethu.reddy@cmich.edu

REFERENCE

1. United Nations. World population ageing 2017 - highlights. Available at: https://www.un.org/en/development/desa/population/publications/pdf/ageing/WPA2017_Highlights.pdf. Accessed June 8, 2020.

Diagnosis of Diabetes Mellitus in Older Adults

S. Sethu K. Reddy, MD, MBA

KEYWORDS

- Diagnosis • Screening • Glucose intolerance • Fasting • Postprandial • OGTT
- HbA1c • Glucose regulation

KEY POINTS

- The burden of diabetes in older adults is steadily increasing in the United States and elsewhere.
- The pathophysiologic factors in the development of type 2 diabetes appear to be exaggerated in older adults.
- Because older adults with diabetes may be asymptomatic, one has to have a high index of suspicion to screen for diabetes.
- One may diagnose diabetes based on globally accepted criteria, relying on fasting glucose values, 2-hour postchallenge results in an oral glucose tolerance test, or on a hemoglobin A1c report.

INTRODUCTION

Diabetes in older adults is an increasingly prevalent clinical challenge.[1] Diabetes is considered the sixth most common cause of death among older adults,[2] but this is likely underestimated because of diabetes not being listed in the 3 causes of death on death certificates.[3] For those who develop diabetes beyond the age of 65 years, life expectancy may be shortened by 4 years.[4] Mortality in older patients with diabetes is strongly correlated with fasting glucose variability and hemoglobin A1c (HbA1c) values.[5] Diabetes in older adults is linked to functional decline and increased health care utilization.[6]

The definition of an older adult is in the eye of the beholder. The World Health Organization (WHO) deems those who are 60 years or older as older,[7] whereas the American Diabetes Association (ADA) defines it as older than 65 years of age,[8] and the International Diabetes Federation considers those over 70 years of age as older.[9] In other spheres, such as human immunodeficiency virus, an older adult is someone who is older than 55 years of age.[10] These criteria are merely a starting point of discussion because one's biological age is more meaningful than chronologic age alone. The prevalence of diabetes in those older than 65 years is close to 20% and increases

CMED 2419, Central Michigan University, Mt. Pleasant, MI 48859, USA
E-mail address: Sethu.reddy@cmich.edu

Clin Geriatr Med 36 (2020) 379–384
https://doi.org/10.1016/j.cger.2020.04.011
0749-0690/20/© 2020 Elsevier Inc. All rights reserved.

with age until 90 years. In long-term care facilities, approximately 25% of residents have diabetes, mostly type 2 diabetes. Of these residents with diabetes, 80% have cardiovascular disease, 56% have hypertension, and 69% have 2 more other chronic conditions. Long-term care residents with diabetes have more falls,[11] higher rates of cardiovascular disease and depression,[12] more functional impairment, and more cognitive decline and dependency than residents without diabetes.[13]

Aging and Changes in Glucose Metabolism

As one ages, there's a tendency to develop more central obesity and thus features suggestive of dysmetabolic syndrome. Glucose regulation changes unfavorably with aging, leading to multifactorial origin of diabetes in older adults. There is dysfunctional insulin secretion and increased resistance to insulin. Increased hepatic glucose production is also observed as one ages. Glucagon secretion in response to hypoglycemia is also impaired.

Rule of thumb

The ability to maintain one's weight, even when obese, is a good indicator of one's persistent insulin secretion capacity.

A family history of diabetes is usually present in those with type 2 diabetes.

Obese individuals (especially central vs peripheral), whose diets are high in saturated fat and low in complex carbohydrates, or who exercise little or are inactive, are more likely to develop diabetes. Tumor necrosis factor-α, produced by adipocytes, is a biomarker highly correlated with insulin resistance and suggests a potential role of inflammation.[14]

Although insulin-mediated glucose uptake is focused on, up to 50% of postprandial glucose uptake may be non–insulin mediated.[15] In the future, non–insulin-mediated glucose uptake could be a target of intervention for diabetes management.

Nutrition: Functional Foods: What Are They?

Recently, there has been a lot of discussion about functional foods (FFs) and diabetes. An FF is a food that is scientifically proven to contribute to improving or preserving the health and well-being and/or reducing the risk of occurrence of diseases related to the diet, beyond its nutrition properties.[16] FFs are part of a normal diet.[17] FFs may thus help prevent and manage chronic diseases, such as type 2 diabetes.[18] FFs may enhance antioxidant, anti-inflammatory, insulin sensitivity, and anticholesterol functions, all quite relevant to diabetes (**Table 1**). The Mediterranean diet is an exemplary

Table 1
Functional foods and potential or proven benefits

Functional Foods	Benefits (Potential/Proven)
Polyunsaturated fatty acids	Vascular health
Plant sterols	Reduce cholesterol levels
Polyphenols (coffee, green tea, black tea)	Vascular health
Probiotic live cultures	Gut health and metabolic effects
Garlic	Anticarcinogenic and anticholesterol
Olive oil	Source of carotenoids
Citrus fruits	Vitamin C
Bananas	Source of potassium
Carrots	Carotenoids

regimen consisting of polyphenols, terpenoids, flavonoids, alkaloids, sterols, pigments, and unsaturated fatty acids.

The full effect of FFs can now be determined by "omics" biological profiling of individuals' molecular, genetics, transcriptomics, proteomics, and metabolomics. Personalized nutrition of the future will no doubt include FFs that are tailored to the patient's needs.

Symptoms of Hyperglycemia in Older Adults

About half of older persons with diabetes will be asymptomatic at the time of diagnosis.[19] An elevated renal threshold for glycosuria in older adults results in absence of polyuria and nocturia, the classic symptoms of diabetes. The thirst mechanism may also be impaired, and the individual can become slowly dehydrated and hyperosmolar. As we age, we also tend to attribute symptoms of fatigue, blurred vision, and numbness to aging itself instead of an organic illness, such as diabetes. Increasingly, diabetes is being diagnosed while one is admitted to a hospital for a nonmetabolic diagnosis, such as myocardial infarction, or elective hip surgery. In long-term care facilities, nonketotic hyperosmolar coma may be the first indication of diabetes.

Depression and hyperglycemia may be associated in a bidirectional manner in older adults. Depression or apparent depression may mask hyperglycemia, and likewise, hyperglycemia causing fatigue and loss of "joie de vivre" may result in false diagnosis of depression.

In many clinics and institutions, it is routine to check fasting glucose levels only. Older adults, in particular,[20] are more likely to have normal fasting glucose levels and abnormally elevated postprandial glucose values.[21] Thus, the diagnosis of diabetes may be missed or delayed. As expected, within long-term care facilities for older adults, those with diabetes have a higher incidence of infections and vascular complications.[22] Macrovascular complications of type 2 diabetes remain the major causes of disability and premature death in older adults with diabetes.[23]

Screening

In the United States, adults older than 65 years of age are eligible to be screened annually for diabetes. The ADA recommends screening all adults older than 45 years of age every 1 to 3 years. The ADA diabetes risk tool suggests that anyone scoring 5 points should be screened.[24] It should be noted that someone 65 years or older starts with 3 points. Thus, it would be very unusual that someone older than 65 years of age would not qualify for diabetes screening.

The diagnosis of diabetes can be made using fasting plasma glucose measurement, with 126 mg/dL (7.0 mmol/L) as the threshold value. Because fasting glucose may be normal in an older adult with diabetes, the WHO has recommended use of the oral glucose tolerance test (OGTT) when possible. A random HbA1c may also be used for diagnosis of diabetes[25]; the advantage of using this biomarker is that the patient need not fast, and the blood sample can be checked at any time of day, because it reflects approximately 3 prior months of glycemic control (**Table 2**).

Older adults are at high risk for both diabetes and prediabetes, with surveillance data suggesting that half of older adults have the latter.[26] The ADA recommends that overweight adults with risk factors, and all adults older than 45 years of age, be screened in the clinical setting every 1 to 3 years, using either fasting plasma glucose, A1C, or OGTT. The recommendations are based on substantial indirect evidence for the benefits of early treatment of type 2 diabetes, the fact that type 2 diabetes is typically undiagnosed for many years, and the knowledge that complications are present at the time of diagnosis.[27]

Table 2
Criteria for diagnosis of prediabetes or diabetes

	Normal	Prediabetes	Diabetes
HbA1c, %	≤5.6	5.7–6.4	≥6.5
Fasting plasma glucose, mg/dL (mmol/L)	≤99 (≤5.5)	100–125 (5.6–6.9)	≥200 (≥11.1)
OGTT (2-h value), mg/dL (mmol/L)	≤139 (≤6.9)	140–199 (7.8–11.0)	≥200 (≥11.1)
Random plasma glucose, mg/dL (mmol/L)	—	—	≥200 (≥11.1)

The benefits of identification of prediabetes and type 2 diabetes in older adults depend on the patient's biological age, patient's life expectancy, and the number of comorbidities. A 67-year-old otherwise healthy individual with type 2 diabetes would warrant more aggressive intervention than an 89-year-old bed-ridden patient with dementia.

The ADA suggests the following parameters:

Symptoms of diabetes plus a casual (any time of day without regard to time since last meal) plasma glucose value of ≥200 mg/dL (≥11.1 mmol/L) (the classic symptoms of diabetes include fatigue, polyuria, polydipsia, and unexplained weight loss); a fasting plasma glucose value of ≥126 mg/dL (≥7.0 mmol/L) (fasting is defined as no caloric intake for at least 8 hours); or a plasma glucose value in the 2-hour sample of the OGTT of ≥200 mg/dL (≥11.1 mmol/L). The test is performed using a load of 75 g of anhydrous glucose.

These criteria reflect an attempt to improve concordance between fasting glucose levels and the 2-hour postglucose levels during OGTT. Also, the risk of macrovascular disease was also taken into account in addition to risk of retinopathy.

It is the author's perspective that OGTT is very useful in the conduct of clinical trials, but for the diagnosis of diabetes in the outpatient setting, one would rely more on the HbA1c measurement in older adults. There is no need to fast, and there is no need for an OGTT for the routine patient.[28]

Rule of thumb
A standardized HbA1c assay is a convenient method to diagnose diabetes mellitus in the older adult.

DISCLOSURE

The author has nothing to disclose.

REFERENCES

1. Laiteerapong N, Huang ES. Diabetes in older adults. Diabetes in America. 3rd edition. Bethesda (MD): National Institutes of Health; 2018. p. 16.

2. Sinclair AJ, Robert IM, Croxson SCM. Mortality in older people with diabetes mellitus. Diabet Med 1996;14:639–47.

3. Meneilly GS, Tessier D. Diabetes in the elderly. In: Morley JE, van den Berg L, editors. Contemporary endocrinology, endocrinology of aging. Totowa (NJ): Humana Press; 2000. p. 181–203.

4. Gu K, Cowie CC, Harris MI. Mortality in adults with and without diabetes in a national cohort of the US population, 1971–1993. Diabetes Care 1998;21:1138–45.
5. Muggeo M, Zoppini G, Bonora E, et al. Fasting plasma glucose variability predicts 10-year survival of type 2 diabetic patients: the Verona Diabetes Study. Diabetes Care 2000;23:45–50.
6. Sari N. Exercise, physical activity and healthcare utilization: a review of literature for older adults. Maturitas 2011;70(3):285–9.
7. World Health Organization. World report on ageing and health. Geneva (Switzerland): World Health Organization; 2015.
8. American Diabetes Association. 12. Older adults: standards of medical care in diabetes—2020. Diabetes Care 2020;43(Supplement 1):S152–62.
9. Dunning T, Sinclair A, Colagiuri S. New IDF guideline for managing type 2 diabetes in older people. Diabetes Res Clin Pract 2014;103(3):538–40.
10. Luther VP, Wilkin AM. HIV infection in older adults. Clin Geriatr Med 2007;23(3): 567–83.
11. Maurer MSBJ, Cheng H. Diabetes mellitus is associated with an increased risk of falls in elderly residents of a long-term care facility. J Gerontol Ser A Biol Sci Med Sci 2005;60:1157–62.
12. Haines ST. The diabetes epidemic: can we stop the spread? Pharmacotherpy 2003;23:1227–31.
13. Travis SS, Buchanan RJ, Wang S, et al. Analyses of nursing home residents with diabetes at admission. J Am Med Dir Assoc 2004;5:320–7.
14. Wu WC, Wei JN, Chen SC, et al. Progression of insulin resistance: a link between risk factors and the incidence of diabetes. Diabetes Res Clin Pract 2020;161: 108050.
15. Best JD, Kahn SE, Ader M, et al. Role of glucose effectiveness in the determination of glucose tolerance. Diabetes Care 1996;19:1018–30.
16. Watson RR. Nutrition and functional foods for healthy aging. Cambridge (MA): Academic Press; 2017.
17. Chiara F, Salvatore FP, Colantuono F, et al. Functional foods for elderly people: new paths for multi "functional" agriculture. Open Agric 2019;4(1):530–43.
18. Alkhatib A, Tsang C, Tiss A, et al. Functional foods and lifestyle approaches for diabetes prevention and management. Nutrients 2017;9(12):1310.
19. Munshi MN, Florez H, Huang ES, et al. Management of diabetes in long-term care and skilled nursing facilities: a position statement of the American Diabetes Association. Diabetes Care 2016;39(2):308–18.
20. Agner E, Thorsteinsson B, Erikson M. Impaired glucose tolerance and diabetes mellitus in elderly subjects. Diabetes Care 1982;5(6):600–4.
21. Monnier L, et al, Monnier L, Colette C. Contributions of fasting and postprandial glucose to hemoglobin A1c. Endocr Pract 2006;12(Supplement 1):42–6.
22. NCD Risk Factor Collaboration, Americas Working Group. Trends in cardiometabolic risk factors in the Americas between 1980 and 2014: a pooled analysis of population-based surveys. Lancet Glob Health 2020;8(1):e123–33.
23. Sloan FA, Bethel MA, Ruiz D, et al. The growing burden of diabetes mellitus in the US elderly population. Arch Intern Med 2008;168(2):192–9.
24. Lindström J, Tuomilehto J. The diabetes risk score: a practical tool to predict type 2 diabetes risk. Diabetes Care 2003;26(3):725–31.
25. Olson DE, Rhee MK, Herrick K, et al. Screening for diabetes and pre-diabetes with proposed A1C-based diagnostic criteria. Diabetes Care 2010;33(10): 2184–9.

26. Centers for Disease Control and Prevention. National diabetes fact sheet: general information and national estimates on diabetes in the United States, 2011. Atlanta (GA): U.S.Department of Health and Human Services, Centers for Disease Control and Prevention; 2011. p. 2011.
27. US Preventive Services Task Force. Screening for type 2 diabetes mellitus in adults: recommendations and rational. Ann Intern Med 2003;138(3):212.
28. World Health Organization. Use of glycated haemoglobin (HbA1c) in diagnosis of diabetes mellitus: abbreviated report of a WHO consultation (No. WHO/NMH/CHP/CPM/11.1). Geneva, Switzerland: World Health Organization; 2011.

Noninsulin Diabetes Therapies in Older Adults

Zehra Tekin, MD, Robert S. Zimmerman, MD*

KEYWORDS

- Diabetes • Older adults • Therapies • Medications • Goal-based algorithm

KEY POINTS

- Elderly adults with type 2 diabetes mellitus need a comprehensive evaluation of medical comorbidities as well as age-related conditions, such as physical or cognitive impairments and financial or personal issues.
- Lifestyle modification recommendations should be individualized but general nutrition and exercise recommendations are similar to those for younger adults.
- Metformin remains the initial choice of pharmacotherapy.
- A goal-based treatment algorithm can be followed when stepping up in medical therapy needed.

INTRODUCTION

Diabetes is one of the most common chronic medical conditions in the elderly population. The prevalence has increased over the past few decades to 1 in every 4 adults ages 65 and older.[1] It has been shown that diabetes in older adults significantly increases morbidity and all-cause mortality compared with the general population.[2] Type 2 diabetes mellitus (T2DM) comprises more than 90% of cases and is thought to be due to age-related defects in β-cell function and increased peripheral insulin resistance.[3,4]

When treating an elderly patient with diabetes, a team-based, patient-centric approach should be used. Patients and families should be provided through education and encouraged to take part in decision making. It has been well documented that collaborative decision making has an impact on glycemic control and disease outcomes.

Although there is substantial heterogeneity in older adults' health and functional capacities, it is known that elderly individuals with diabetes are at high risk for vascular diseases, such as coronary artery disease, as well as physical and

Endocrinology, Diabetes and Metabolism Institute, Cleveland Clinic Foundation, 9500 Euclid Avenue, F-20, Cleveland, OH 44195, USA
* Corresponding author.
E-mail address: zimmerr@ccf.org

0749-0690/20/© 2020 Elsevier Inc. All rights reserved.

cognitive impairments.[5] Treatment choices should be made while considering patients' age, cognitive function, diabetes duration and complications, comorbid illnesses, and psychosocial and financial issues as well as personal beliefs and preferences.

Diabetes management requires intact cognitive function to fully execute self-care activities, including maintaining a healthy diet, self-monitoring of blood glucose (SMBG), and medication and insulin administration as well as hypoglycemia or hyperglycemia management. Self-care can become challenging for individuals with cognitive decline and may cause the failure of treatment or suboptimal glycemic control because it has been shown that the presence of cognitive impairment in patients with diabetes increases both hypoglycemia and hyperglycemia risk.[6,7] Therefore, it is imperative to obtain a full assessment of patients' cognitive abilities and clinical conditions at first visit followed by screenings at regular intervals with available tools, such as Montreal Cognitive Assessment, Mini-Cog, and Mini-Mental State Examination.[8–10] Cognitive assessment also should be done whenever diabetes control worsens unexpectedly or if glycemic targets are not achieved. Patients who are identified to have cognitive issues should be referred to appropriate providers, such as geriatricians, neurologists, and/or psychiatrists, for definitive evaluation. Treatment regimens should be kept as simple as possible in these individuals to increase adherence and avoid hypoglycemia.

Patients' adherence to treatment should be assessed regularly with a nonjudgmental approach and any barriers to compliance need to be addressed vigilantly. Physicians also should collaborate with families or caregivers to identify potential issues for successful disease management. Continuing patient and family education is considered key to preventing acute and long-term complications of diabetes (see Khine Swe and S. Sethu Reddy's article, Improving Adherence in Type 2 Diabetes," in this issue).

Psychosocial problems, such as anxiety, depression, loss of autonomy and dependability, lack of social networks, and financial constraints also commonly are seen in the elderly population and should be addressed as part of comprehensive diabetes care.[11] Validated screenings for depression, such as the Geriatric Depression Scale, Hamilton Depression Rating Scale, and Patient Health Questionnaire-9, can be used.[12–14]

Physical impairments seen in the elderly population, such as vision or hearing loss and difficulty ambulating, can worsen disease control significantly, so they need to be assessed in each patient, and treatment regimen should be tailored accordingly.[15]

Another important issue to keep in mind in the elderly population is polypharmacy.[16] Due to an increased number of medications, older adults are prone to having problems with adherence and side effects, including falls.[17] An inverse correlation has been established between the number of medications and the frequency of administration and medication compliance.[18]

Because hypoglycemia is a common problem that occurs in older adults due to blunted counter-regulatory responses as well as a result of a decline in renal function and cognitive impairment, the authors recommend that medications that are known to increase the risk of hypoglycemia be avoided.[19] This issue is addressed in Beers Criteria for Potentially Inappropriate Medication Use in Older Adults, commonly called the Beers List, which is an evidence-based guideline released by the American Geriatrics Society.[20] The latest version of the list was released in 2019, with updated recommendations for diabetes medications, mainly due to the risk of hypoglycemia, which should be taken into consideration. **Table 1** shows antihyperglycemic noninsulin agents included in the Beers List.

Table 1
Antihyperglycemic noninsulin agents included in the 2019 beers criteria for potentially inappropriate medication use in older adults

Agent	Recommendation	Quality of Evidence	Strength of Evidence	Rationale

• SUs, long acting
  • Chlorpropamide
  • Glimepiride*
  • Glyburide
    (also known as
    glibenclamide)
	Avoid	High	Strong	Chlorpropamide: prolonged half-life in older adults; can cause prolonged hypoglycemia; causes syndrome of inappropriate antidiuretic hormone secretion
				Glimepiride and glyburide: higher risk of severe prolonged hypoglycemia in older adults

* newly added. *Adapted from* Fick DM, Semla TP, Steinman M, et al. American Geriatrics Society 2019 updated AGS Beers Criteria® for potentially inappropriate medication use in older adults. J Am Geriatr Soc. 2019;67(4):674-694; with permission.

COMPREHENSIVE MEDICAL EVALUATION AND GLYCEMIC TARGETS

Given the increased number of chronic medical conditions, mainly cardiovascular and renal diseases by age, a comprehensive medical evaluation should be made when treating older adults with T2DM.[21] Glycemic targets must be individualized according to comorbid illnesses. Based on patients' overall clinical condition and diabetes complications, a hemoglobin A_{1c} goal can range from less than 7.5% in otherwise healthy older adults to less than 8.5% in patients with multiple complications or severe cognitive impairment.[21]

Hemoglobin A_{1c} levels should be correlated with patient SMBG data because there can be discrepancies due to excursions of blood sugar or comorbid conditions affecting red cell life span, such as anemia, renal failure, and recent blood transfusions.[22] Continuous glucose monitoring should be used in older adults who have inconsistent hemoglobin A_{1c} levels and SMBG data.[23]

LIFESTYLE MODIFICATIONS
Nutrition

Regardless of age, healthy diet modifications are one of the most impactful lifestyle interventions recommended to achieve glycemic targets for patients with T2DM as part of disease self-management.[24]

Older adults may have particular challenges in following the recommendations of clinicians for a variety of reasons, including decreased financial resources or disability limiting their chance for shopping or preparing food. Cognitive impairment also can lead to malnutrition in this population. They also may have other issues, such as a change in sense of taste or poor dentition, affecting their oral intake. Therefore, the authors recommend that older adults with T2DM be evaluated by a Registered Dietitian and/or a Certified Diabetes Educator for detailed education and development of individual nutrition planning. It also is critically important to assess patients' personal preferences, eating habits, and financial abilities before making recommendations.

There are no special recommendations for macronutrient distribution in older adults, but heart-healthy diets rich in protein content can be encouraged to avoid sarcopenia because there is an age-related decline in lean body mass.

Fluid intake may not be optimal in elderly adults due to mobility issues and decreased thirst sensation. Elderly adults should be encouraged to maintain good hydration to avoid the risk of hyperosmolar hyperglycemic nonketotic syndrome, unless it is contraindicated otherwise due to other coexisting diseases, such as heart or renal failure.

Physical Activity

Daily physical activity has important benefits in patients with T2DM at any age because exercise increases insulin sensitivity, promotes weight loss, maintains physical condition, and improves overall glycemic control. The American Diabetes Association recommendations are similar to those for the younger adults and include 30 minutes of moderate-intensity aerobic activity (eg, brisk walking) at least 5 days per week and muscle-strengthening activities 2 days each week.[25]

Exercise should be individualized based on patients' fall risk and level of physical impairment because older adults with T2DM are known to have a higher risk of falls compared with the same age group of patients without diabetes. Patients who are considered to be at high risk can be referred to an exercise physiologist and/or physical therapist for further evaluation.

MEDICATIONS
Metformin

Metformin is a biguanide that has long been in use as the first-line pharmacotherapy for the treatment of T2DM. It reduces hepatic glucose output and enhances insulin sensitivity with resultant hemoglobin A_{1c} reduction of approximately 1.5%.[26] Metformin remains as the initial therapeutic choice in patients ages 65 years and older with diabetes in addition to lifestyle management due to its efficacy and potential for modest weight loss without having the risk of hypoglycemia.[27] Unfortunately, there are few randomized controlled trials specially designed for older adults to date to evaluate oral antihyperglycemic agents. The UK Prospective Diabetes Study, which was the first large-scale study to demonstrate a substantial cardiovascular benefit of metformin, with a 36% relative risk reduction in all-cause mortality and a 39% relative risk reduction in myocardial infarction, has enrolled mainly middle-aged subjects with new onset of disease and has excluded patients above the age of 65.[28]

Metformin use is contraindicated in patients with renal failure, with estimated glomerular filtration rate of 30 mL/min/1.73 m^2 or less, or who have gastrointestinal intolerance. Although considered a rare side effect, with the incidence of less than 1 case per 100,000 treated patients, lactic acidosis can occur in certain conditions, such as acute kidney injury, heart failure, or radiocontrast dye use. Due to the uncertainty of a patient's clinical course, metformin also is recommended to be held in hospitalized patients. Vitamin B_{12} deficiency is seen more commonly in elderly adults due to changes in diet and can be precipitated by prolonged metformin use; therefore, annual monitoring of serum levels is recommended.

Sulfonylureas and Meglitinides

Sulfonylureas (SUs) work on receptors that block the adenosine triphosphate–sensitive potassium channels in pancreatic β cells, which causes cells to depolarize and triggers the cascade of insulin secretion.[29] Repaglinide and nateglinide are meglitinides (also known as glinides), which are structurally different but act similarly to SUs by binding to the same receptor, although with lower affinity.[30] They have a shorter duration of action and are used at mealtimes to treat postprandial hyperglycemia. Both classes reduce hemoglobin A_{1c} between 1% and 1.5% and generally are inexpensive but are associated with potential prolonged hypoglycemia and weight gain (see Byron J. Hoogwerf's article, "Hypoglycemia in the Older Patient," in this issue).

As listed in the Beers criteria, long-acting SUs and glyburide should be avoided in older individuals because of markedly increased risk of hypoglycemia. Other SUs can be considered for patients with financial constraints and difficult to control diabetes. Extensive counseling and education should be done prior to initiation of therapy and the patients who are on SUs need more frequent blood sugar monitoring.

Thiazolidinediones

Thiazolidinediones (TZDs), or glitazones, exert their peripheral effects on a nuclear receptor, peroxisome proliferator-activated receptor-γ, triggering a cascade to increase insulin sensitivity.[31] TZDs, mainly pioglitazone and rosiglitazone, reduce hemoglobin A_{1c} by 0.5% to 1% without risk of hypoglycemia. Although proved to have modest cardiovascular benefits, their use is limited due to weight gain and fluid retention. It also has been shown that TZDs increase bone loss and fracture risk in women, which increases the risk of osteoporosis in older adults.

α-Glucosidase Inhibitors

α-Glucosidase inhibitors work locally in the small intestine by blocking the breakdown of oligosaccharides, trisaccharides, and disaccharides, which in turn reduces the absorption of carbohydrates, resulting in a modest reduction in postprandial blood sugars with hemoglobin A_{1c} reduction of approximately 0.5% to 1.0%.[32] The use of these agents is limited, mainly due to their modest efficacy and lower tolerability due to gastrointestinal side effects, including flatulence and diarrhea. Patients who use these agents should be counseled to treat any hypoglycemia with glucose tablets, which are monosaccharides, rather than sucrose (table sugar, juices, and so forth), because the breakdown of sucrose is inhibited by this medication.

Dipeptidyl Peptidase-4 Inhibitors

Incretins, such as glucagon-like peptide 1 (GLP-1) and glucose-dependent insulinotropic peptide, lower blood sugars via several mechanisms, including increased glucose-dependent insulin secretion, decreased glucagon levels, delayed gastric emptying, and induction of satiety.[33] Dipeptidyl peptidase (DPP)-4 inhibitors, or gliptin, block the enzyme responsible from inactivation and degradation of incretins and reduce hemoglobin A_{1c} by 0.5% to 1.0%, with no risk of weight gain or hypoglycemia.

Although DPP-4 inhibitors have been reported to have a neutral cardiovascular effect, there is reportedly increased risk of admission for heart failure with use of saxagliptin and alogliptin. This class of medication generally is well tolerated. There has been some association of pancreatitis and idiopathic arthralgia but no cause-effect relationship is evident.

Sodium-Glucose Cotransporter 2 Inhibitors

Sodium-glucose cotransporter 2 (SGLT2) inhibitors, or gliflozins, are recently approved by the Food and Drug Administration for use in patients with diabetes. The class works by inhibiting sodium-glucose transport protein 2, which reabsorbs glucose from the kidney; thereby, facilitating urinary excretion of excess glucose and lowering hemoglobin A_{1c} by approximately 0.8% to 1%.[34]

SGLT2 inhibitors also mediate renal sodium reabsorption; thus, inhibition leads to changes in fluid balance, and beneficial effects observed in heart failure patients in reducing hospitalization for heart failure exacerbation. Besides, these agents have been found to decrease renal complications of diabetes and also are associated with a modest weight reduction.

SHLT2 inhibitors have been reported to be associated with an increased incidence of both urinary tract infections and genital tract infections as well as volume depletion and decrease in bone mineral density. Although rare, there are cases with euglycemic ketoacidosis reported in patients with T2DM who are using these agents.

Glucagon-Like Peptide 1 Receptor Agonists

Incretins have been studied for decades due to their previously discussed effects in glucose homeostasis[33] before the first GLP-1 receptor agonists became clinically available in the United States in 2005. The class has been showed to have beneficial cardiovascular effects and is favored in obese patients due to their weight loss effects.[35] They have been showed to increase the risk of pancreatitis and carry a black box warning for the risk of medullary thyroid carcinoma. A limitation to their use has been their route of administration (subcutaneous injection). The Food and Drug Administration recently approved the first oral form of GLP-1 receptor agonists in September 2019. Another issue is tolerability due to gastrointestinal side effects, mainly nausea and diarrhea.

Amylin Agonists

Amylin is a hormone that is cosecreted with insulin from pancreatic βcells in response to meal intake. It delays gastric emptying and decreases glucagon secretion and also works in the brain and suppresses appetite.[36] Amylin analogs are approved for the treatment of both type 1 diabetes mellitus and T2DM. These agents are administered subcutaneously with meals and improve postprandial glycemic excursions with a modest reduction in hemoglobin A_{1c} (<1%) with favorable effects on weight. Common side effects of amylin analogs include nausea, vomiting, decreased appetite, headaches, and hypoglycemia, especially when used in conjunction with insulin. The need for 3 injections per day has limited the utilization of these agents.

Bromocriptine

Quick-release bromocriptine is a dopamine receptor agonist that is administered orally within 2 hours of awakening and has been shown to re-establish morning brain dopamine D2 receptor activity, which reduces sympathetic tone, resulting in increased insulin sensitivity and decreased blood sugars with overall hemoglobin A_{1c} reductions approximately 0.5% to 0.7%.[37] Common side effects include nausea, fatigue, dizziness, vomiting, and headache.

Patients should also be warned about possible psychotic adverse events, although these usually are seen with the use of higher doses.

Colesevelam

Colesevelam is a second-generation bile acid sequestrant that has been shown to improve blood glucose levels in patients with diabetes with a modest reduction in hemoglobin A_{1c} approximately 0.5%.[38] Due to limited clinical experience and cost, it is not been widely used. Common side effects include constipation, nausea, and dyspepsia.

GOAL-BASED THERAPY

Older adults with diabetes who do not reach glycemic targets with lifestyle interventions and metformin alone should add other oral or injectable agents and/or insulin to their regimen.[39] The American Diabetes Association recommends following a goal-based algorithm, which allows the physician to identify the patient goals and pick agents that best support these goals while considering glycemic control, cardiovascular benefits, avoidance of hypoglycemia, promotion of weight loss or neutrality, and affordability for the patient (**Fig. 1**).

As discussed previously, when choosing a second-line agent for older adults with diabetes who are at high risk of hypoglycemia, it is recommended that insulin secretagogues, such as SUs, and exogenous insulin therapy are avoided as much as possible.

When weight control is desired, agents that cause weight loss, such as GLP-1 analogs or SGLT-2 inhibitors, provide the best outcomes, whereas DPP-4 inhibitors are weight neutral. Weight gain is associated with sulfonylureas, TZDs, and insulin and therefore are not recommended in these patients.

For patients with established cardiovascular disease, SGLT2 inhibitors or GLP-1 analogs with proved cardiovascular benefits are recommended as second-line agents.[40] SGLT2 inhibitors should be favored in patients with established heart failure or renal disease (as glomerular filtration rate allows).

If financial limitations exist, SUs and TZDs can be used.

Initiation of dual oral therapy should be considered in older adults who are newly diagnosed with T2DM and have hemoglobin A_{1c} more than 8.5% to 9% and insulin therapy when hemoglobin A_{1c} is significantly elevated (>10% [86 mmol/mol]) or blood

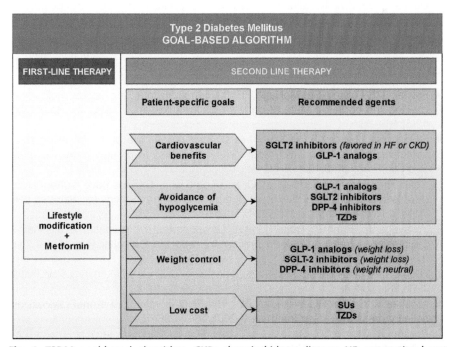

Fig. 1. T2DM goal-based algorithm. CKD, chronic kidney disease; HF, congestive heart failure.

glucose levels are very high ($\geq$300 mg/dL [16.7 mmol/L]).[41] Diabetes regimen should be monitored every 3 months to 6 months and intensified as needed after reviewing the potential barriers to achieving target glycemic control.

DISCLOSURE

Dr Z. Tekin has nothing to disclose. Dr R.S. Zimmerman is a speaker for Merck and Lifescan.

REFERENCES

1. National diabetes statistics report, 2017. Atlanta (GA): Centers for Disease Control US Dept Heal Hum Serv; 2017.
2. Bertoni AG, Krop JS, Anderson GF, et al. Diabetes-related morbidity and mortality in a national sample of U.S. elders. Diabetes Care 2002;25(3):471–5.
3. Laiteerapong N, Karter AJ, Liu JY, et al. Correlates of quality of life in older adults with diabetes: the diabetes & aging study. Diabetes Care 2011;34(8):1749–53.
4. Huang ES, Laiteerapong N, Liu JY, et al. Rates of complications and mortality in older patients with diabetes mellitus: the diabetes and aging study. JAMA Intern Med 2014;174(2):251–8.
5. Ott A, Stolk RP, Van Harskamp F, et al. Diabetes mellitus and the risk of dementia: the Rotterdam Study. Neurology 1999;53(9):1937–42.
6. De Galan BE, Zoungas S, Chalmers J, et al. Cognitive function and risks of cardiovascular disease and hypoglycaemia in patients with type 2 diabetes: the action in diabetes and vascular disease: preterax and diamicron modified release controlled evaluation (ADVANCE) trial. Diabetologia 2009;52(11):2328–36.
7. Davydow DS, Zivin K, Katon WJ, et al. Neuropsychiatric disorders and potentially preventable hospitalizations in a prospective cohort study of older americans. J Gen Intern Med 2014;29(10):1362–71.
8. Nasreddine ZS, Phillips NA, BÃ©dirian V, et al. The Montreal cognitive assessment, MoCA: a brief screening tool for mild cognitive impairment. J Am Geriatr Soc 2005;53(4):695–9.
9. Folstein MF, Folstein SE, McHugh PR. "Mini-mental state". A practical method for grading the cognitive state of patients for the clinician. J Psychiatr Res 1975; 12(3):189–98.
10. Sinclair AJ, Gadsby R, Hillson R, et al. Brief report: use of the Mini-Cog as a screening tool for cognitive impairment in diabetes in primary care. Diabetes Res Clin Pract 2013;100(1):e23–5.
11. Chau PH, Woo J, Lee CH, et al. Older people with diabetes have higher risk of depression, cognitive and functional impairments: implications for diabetes services. J Nutr Health Aging 2011;15(9):751–5.
12. Yesavage JA, Brink TL, Rose TL, et al. Development and validation of a geriatric depression screening scale: a preliminary report. J Psychiatr Res 1982;17(1): 37–49.
13. HAMILTON M. A rating scale for depression. J Neurol Neurosurg Psychiatry 1960;23(1):56–62.
14. Kroenke K, Spitzer RL, Williams JBW. The PHQ-9: validity of a brief depression severity measure. J Gen Intern Med 2001;16(9):606–13.
15. Bossoni S, Mazziotti G, Gazzaruso C, et al. Relationship between instrumental activities of daily living and blood glucose control in elderly subjects with type 2 diabetes [4]. Age Ageing 2008;37(2):222–5.

16. Linjakumpu T, Hartikainen S, Klaukka T, et al. Use of medications and polypharmacy are increasing among the elderly. J Clin Epidemiol 2002;55(8):809–17.

17. Sergi G, De Rui M, Sarti S, et al. Polypharmacy in the elderly: can comprehensive geriatric assessment reduce inappropriate medication use? Drugs Aging 2011; 28(7):509–18.

18. Claxton AJ, Cramer J, Pierce C. A systematic review of the associations between dose regimens and medication compliance. Clin Ther 2001;23(8):1296–310.

19. Alagiakrishnan K, Mereu L. Approach to managing hypoglycemia in older adults with diabetes. Postgrad Med 2010;122(3):129–37.

20. Fick DM, Semla TP, Steinman M, et al. American Geriatrics Society 2019 Updated AGS beers criteria® for potentially inappropriate medication use in older adults. J Am Geriatr Soc 2019;67(4):674–94.

21. Kirkman MS, Briscoe VJ, Clark N, et al. Diabetes in older adults. Diabetes Care 2012;35(12):2650–64.

22. Gallagher EJ, Le Roith D, Bloomgarden Z. Review of hemoglobin A1c in the management of diabetes. J Diabetes 2009;1(1):9–17.

23. Danne T, Nimri R, Battelino T, et al. International consensus on use of continuous glucose monitoring. Diabetes Care 2017;40(12):1631–40.

24. Redmond EH, Burnett SM, Johnson MA, et al. Improvement in A1C levels and diabetes self-management activities following a nutrition and diabetes education program in older adults. J Nutr Elder 2007;26(1–2):83–102.

25. Colberg SR, Sigal RJ, Yardley JE, et al. Physical activity/exercise and diabetes: a position statement of the American Diabetes Association. Diabetes Care 2016; 39(11):2065–79.

26. Defronzo RA, Goodman AM. Efficacy of metformin in patients with non-insulin-dependent diabetes mellitus. N Engl J Med 1995;333(9):541–9.

27. Viollet B, Guigas B, Sanz Garcia N, et al. Cellular and molecular mechanisms of metformin: an overview. Clin Sci 2012;122(6):253–70.

28. Turner R. Effect of intensive blood-glucose control with metformin on complications in overweight patients with type 2 diabetes (UKPDS 34). Lancet 1998; 352(9131):854–65.

29. Aguilar-Bryan L, Nichols CG, Wechsler SW, et al. Cloning of the β cell high-affinity sulfonylurea receptor: a regulator of insulin secretion. Science 1995;268(5209): 423–6.

30. Fuhlendorff J, Rorsman P, Kofod H, et al. Stimulation of insulin release by repaglinide and glibenclamide involves both common and distinct processes. Diabetes 1998;47(3):345–51.

31. Nolan JJ, Ludvik B, Beerdsen P, et al. Improvement in glucose tolerance and insulin resistance in obese subjects treated with troglitazone. N Engl J Med 1994; 331(18):1188–93.

32. Hoffmann J, Spengler M. Efficacy of 24-week monotherapy with acarbose, glibenclamide, or placebo in NIDDM patients: the essen study. Diabetes Care 1994;17(6):561–6.

33. Baggio LL, Drucker DJ. Biology of incretins: GLP-1 and GIP. Gastroenterology 2007;132(6):2131–57.

34. Vasilakou D, Karagiannis T, Athanasiadou E, et al. Sodium-glucose cotransporter 2 inhibitors for type 2 diabetes: a systematic review and meta-analysis. Ann Intern Med 2013;159(4):262–74.

35. Zander M, Madsbad S, Madsen JL, et al. Effect of 6-week course of glucagon-like peptide 1 on glycaemic control, insulin sensitivity, and β-cell function in type 2 diabetes: a parallel-group study. Lancet 2002;359(9309):824–30.

36. Whitehouse F, Kruger DF, Fineman M, et al. A randomized study and open-label extension evaluating the long-term efficacy of pramlintide as an adjunct to insulin therapy in type 1 diabetes. Diabetes Care 2002;25(4):724–30.

37. Kamath V, Jones CN, Yip JC, et al. Effects of a quick-release form of bromocriptine (Ergoset) on fasting and postprandial plasma glucose, insulin, lipid, and lipoprotein concentrations in obese nondiabetic hyperinsulinemic women. Diabetes Care 1997;20(11):1697–701.

38. Ooi CP, Loke SC. Colesevelam for type 2 diabetes mellitus. Cochrane Database Syst Rev 2012;2017(12). https://doi.org/10.1002/14651858.CD009361.pub2.

39. American Diabetes Association. 12. Older adults: standards of medical care in diabetes—2019. Diabetes Care 2018;42(Supplement 1):S139–47.

40. Sarafidis P, Ferro CJ, Morales E, et al. SGLT-2 inhibitors and GLP-1 receptor agonists for nephroprotection and cardioprotection in patients with diabetes mellitus and chronic kidney disease. A consensus statement by the EURECA-m and the DIABESITY working groups of the ERA-EDTA. Nephrol Dial Transplant 2019; 34(2):208–30.

41. American Diabetes Association. 9. Pharmacologic approaches to glycemic treatment: standards of medical care in diabetes—2019. Diabetes Care 2019; 42(Supplement 1):S90–102.

Hypoglycemia in Older Patients

Byron J. Hoogwerf, MD[a,b,*]

KEYWORDS

- Diabetes mellitus • Elderly • Hyperglycemia • Hypoglycemia • Older patients

KEY POINTS

- Glucose control with medications is associated with a risk for hypoglycemia.
- Multiple risk factors, including medications and associated medical conditions, increase hypoglycemia risk.
- Older patients may be at greater risk for adverse outcomes associated with hypoglycemia.
- Glycemic targets may need to be adjusted in older patients to reduce hypoglycemia risk.
- Cognitive dysfunction, hypoglycemic unawareness, and medical comorbidities require appropriate education by the health care team.

INTRODUCTION

Although diabetes mellitus (DM) has been known for several millennia, the concept of hypoglycemia is less than a century old. Hypoglycemia was first noted with the use of the pancreatic extract that came to be known as insulin. Robert Tattersall's[1] comprehensive work on diabetes elegantly describes the early observations in which normal rabbits injected with insulin sometimes developed convulsions and a young boy became comatose with insulin use.[1] Each of these events was remedied by glucose. These early "protean manifestations" (Tattersall's[1] term) of insulin-induced hypoglycemia were not deemed to be serious because of the rapid responses to intravenous glucose.

Over the past century the understanding of the seriousness of hypoglycemia and factors associated with hypoglycemia, including compromise of quality of life, potential for serious neurologic damage, and associations with cardiovascular disease (CVD) risk, have been the focus of much investigation. Furthermore, there is evidence that the early adrenergic/autonomic responses that help patients identify evolving hypoglycemia may be lost, resulting in hypoglycemic unawareness and the attendant increased risk for severe hypoglycemia.[2,3] Hypoglycemic unawareness has had

[a] Cleveland Clinic, Cleveland, OH, USA; [b] Central Michigan University, College of Medicine, Mount Pleasant, MI, USA
* 8972 Huntington Pointe Drive, Sarasota, FL 34238.
E-mail address: byronhoogwerf@gmail.com

Clin Geriatr Med 36 (2020) 395–406
https://doi.org/10.1016/j.cger.2020.04.001
0749-0690/20/© 2020 Elsevier Inc. All rights reserved.

geriatric.theclinics.com

significant impact on the management of hyperglycemia, especially in the selection of glucose lowering agents and advances in the ability of patients to monitor their own blood glucose levels.[3] Each of these considerations is important to aging/older/elderly patients with DM.

This article focuses on information obtained in older patients. Studies that were not limited to older patients are included when the data are likely applicable to older patients. At the outset it should be noted that, in many trials and observational datasets, elderly is often defined as age greater than 65 years. Although this age is lower than many conventional clinical definitions used in geriatrics, this cutoff is used because of the volume of data using it. In addition, there are 5 generally accepted definitions of hypoglycemia: severe hypoglycemia (requires assistance); documented symptomatic hypoglycemia; asymptomatic hypoglycemia; probable symptomatic hypoglycemia; pseudohypoglycemia (symptoms, but blood glucose level >70 mg/dL).[3] In most of the reports cited here, severe hypoglycemia is the commonest definition used, although in some cases documented symptomatic hypoglycemia is also evaluated.

Glycemic Management Guidelines and the Magnitude of Hypoglycemia Risk

Guidelines for the management of hyperglycemia have usually focused on glycemic targets such as hemoglobin A1c (HbA1c).[4–8] At the outset it should be noted that, if an older adult gets to an HbA1c level of 7% without any hypoglycemia with a simple antihyperglycemic regimen, then there is no need to reduce medical therapy. However, clinicians should not be needlessly aggressive with target achievement and put the patient at risk of hypoglycemia. Over the past 10 years, there has been increased recognition that glycemic targets should be adjusted to higher levels in older and more vulnerable patients. Observations from large cardiovascular outcomes trials in which little CVD benefit was observed and hypoglycemia was associated with adverse outcomes were at the core of these recommendations.[9] Ismail-Beigi and colleagues[9] reviewed these data and recommended that higher HbA1c levels were appropriate for older patients, and these recommendations were incorporated into guidelines.[5] These recommendations are driven by the fact that hypoglycemia in older patients poses risks that are likely greater than in younger patients. Tseng and colleagues[10] studied a large (>2 million) Veterans' Affairs population in which more than 25% of patients on sulfonylureas and/or insulin were aged 75 years and older, of whom more than half on insulin and/or sulfonylureas had HbA1c levels less than 7.0%. Andrews and O'Malley[11] in an accompanying editorial note: "Given the risks associated with intensive glycemic control in elderly individuals and in those with chronic medical conditions, it now behooves physicians and health systems to understand the extent of potential diabetic overtreatment in everyday practice and seek to improve it." In a more recent observational study from Kaiser of Northern California, Weiner and colleagues[12] reported that insulin was more likely to be continued in patients with more comorbid conditions and discontinued in healthier older patients. In the context of these observations, this article seeks to characterize features associated with hypoglycemia in older patients and clinical considerations in managing hypoglycemia risk in older patients with DM.

HYPOGLYCEMIA IN OLDER PATIENTS: ADVERSE EFFECTS, RISK FACTORS, AND DETECTION
Quality of Life

Several features of hypoglycemia contribute to the potential for compromised quality of life. If a patient has had a hypoglycemic reaction, there is always the fear of another episode. Hypoglycemia is often detected by others who live with the person with DM, but older patients are often spouseless and thus are deprived of an important hypoglycemia detection support. For patients who take insulin or sulfonylureas, the need to eat on a regular schedule may limit the lifestyle flexibility that people without DM may enjoy. A serious hypoglycemic reaction that results in a motor vehicle accident may result in the loss of driving privileges, further compromising activities of daily living.

Cognitive Impairment

Hypoglycemia may contribute to acute cognitive impairment in any patient with DM. This impairment occurs because the brain is an obligate glucose user and neuroglycopenia affects cognitive function. In older patients who already have some memory loss, cognitive impairment associated with hypoglycemia may go unrecognized. Recurrent hypoglycemia has been associated with increased risk for cognitive decline. Whether this is a direct effect of hypoglycemia or the fact that hypoglycemia risk and the need for insulin both increase as a function of duration of DM is still uncertain. A relationship between hypoglycemia and cognitive impairment was concisely summarized by Umegaki and colleagues[13]: "Cognitive impairment which often exists with frailty syndrome has a bidirectional association with hypoglycemia. Cognitive impairment is a risk for hypoglycemia, and hypoglycemia induces cognitive impairment."

Frailty and Falls

Frailty as defined by standard clinical criteria not only increases with age but is higher in older patients with DM.[13–15] Hypoglycemia predisposes to the risk for falls because of associated lack of coordination and cognitive dysfunction, often aggravated by medication use.[16,17] This risk occurs in any patient with hypoglycemia. Because falls are an aging-associated risk, this risk is increased in the elderly.

Counter-Regulatory Hormone and Symptomatic Responses to Hypoglycemia in Older Patients

Older patients have evidence of an impaired counter-regulatory response to hypoglycemia. Whether this is a result of the altered counter-regulatory responses as originally reported from Cryer's group[2] or whether there is altered ability to detect hypoglycemia for some other reason is not entirely clear. Meneilly and colleagues[18] studied 10 healthy patients and 10 patients with type 2 DM with a mean age of 74 years. In hypoglycemic clamp studies, mean glucagon and growth hormone responses were lower in the patients with DM. However, epinephrine and cortisol levels were higher. Hypoglycemic symptoms were comparable in both groups.[18] By contrast, Bremer and colleagues[19] reported no differences in hormonal responses between older and middle-aged subjects, but clinical detection of autonomic and neuroglycopenic symptoms was impaired in the older patients.

Variables Associated with Hypoglycemia Risk

There are multiple studies that have looked for associations or risk factors for hypoglycemia (**Box 1**).[2,16,19–39] Four large studies serve to set the stage for key variables associated with hypoglycemia. Pathak and colleagues[20] reported one of the largest epidemiologic studies in 917,440 patients with DM in whom the severe hypoglycemia rate was 1.4 to 1.6 events per 100 person years. Rates of severe hypoglycemia were higher with older age; chronic kidney disease; congestive heart failure (HF); CVD; depression; higher HbA1c levels; and in users of insulin, insulin

---

Box 1
Risk factors associated with hypoglycemia in older patients with diabetes mellitus

Increasing age

Increasing duration of DM

Medications
    Glucose level lowering: insulin, sulfonylureas, short-acting insulin secretagogues
    β-Blockers
    Angiotensin-converting enzyme inhibitors
    Ethanol

Medical conditions
    Chronic renal failure
    Hepatic dysfunction
    Cardiovascular disease
    Heart failure
    Cognitive dysfunction
    Sarcopenia/frailty

---

secretagogues, or β -blockers. Hypoglycemia rate in persons aged 70 to 84 years was 2.55 events per 100 person years and, for persons aged 85 years or older, was 2.81. The highest rates were in patients taking long-acting insulin (3.18 events per 100 person years) and short-acting insulin (5.03 per 100 person years). For other comorbidities, the rates were 5.26 for CKD, 7.19 for CHF, and 5.37 for the CVD cohort. In this cohort, the risk was 2.58 for HbA1c levels greater than or equal to 9.0% compared with 0.96 for HbA1c levels less than 7.0%. These associations are similar to those reported by others. However, other studies report an increased risk for hypoglycemia associated with lower HbA1c level. This disparity may be partially addressed with the following considerations. On one hand, patients with lower HbA1c levels have glucose levels that are generally closer to the hypoglycemic thresholds. By contrast, with longer duration of disease, HbA1c levels are higher, there is greater glucose variability, more comorbidities, and greater use of insulin. Efforts to aggressively reduce HbA1c levels, especially with insulin, may contribute to the greater risk for hypoglycemia in spite of higher HbA1c levels. The Action to Control Cardiovascular Risk in Diabetes (ACCORD) trial was a specific example in which intensification to achieve a target HbA1c level of less than 6.0% showed that patients with the highest HbA1c values had the highest risk for severe hypoglycemia. Although ACCORD was not performed specifically in an older population, the analyses of risk factors associated with severe hypoglycemia by Miller and colleagues[21] are instructive. When hypoglycemia requiring assistance was analyzed for the whole cohort, the following hazard ratios were statistically significant: age (per 1-year increase), 1.03; serum creatinine level greater than 114.9 μmol/L (vs <88.4 μmol/L), 1.66; time since diagnosis of DM (16+ years vs ≤5 years), 1.37. Increased body weight was associated with a reduced risk for hypoglycemia (body mass index ≥30 vs <25): 0.65. Risk of hypoglycemia related to insulin use and HbA1c were analyzed in both the intensive and conventional treatment groups. In the conventional arm, being on any insulin had a hazard ratio (HR) of 4.08 and, in the intensive group, an HR of 1.95. Increased HbA1c level was associated with increased hypoglycemia risk, with an HR of 1.3 for every 1% increase in HbA1c level. No association of HbA1c level and hypoglycemia risk was seen in the intensive group. Of note, there was no association with CVD, but this was a cohort characterized by high CVD risk, so no comparison with a truly low-risk group was possible.

The Pathak and colleagues[20] and ACCORD datasets both show that age, renal disease, and insulin use are associated with increased hypoglycemia risk. These studies are representative of many other datasets from both observational cohorts and randomized clinical trials. The observation that increasing weight is associated with less hypoglycemia[21] may be important for the elderly, in whom lower weight and sarcopenia may characterize an at-risk patient cohort for hypoglycemia.

Fu and colleagues[22] analyzed hypoglycemia-related hospitalizations using a database of 887,182 people with type 2 DM. The most important risk factor for hypoglycemia hospitalizations was age. In a methodology in which all contributors to hypoglycemia add to 100%, age more than 65 years contributed 31.17%, followed by sulfonylurea use (30.03%), insulin use (13.49%), and renal disease (8.29%). In patients more than 65 years of age, the greatest risks for hypoglycemia hospitalizations were use of insulin plus sulfonylurea, insulin use, sulfonylurea use, renal disease, and a prior hospitalization for hypoglycemia event. These observations are corroborated by such studies as those reported by Bramlage and colleagues,[23] who performed an observational cohort study of 3810 patients with DM in which 1373 patients aged greater than 70 years had more hypoglycemia than the 1233 patients aged less than 60 years. In addition to sulfonylurea use, stroke/transitory ischemic attacks, HF, and depression were all more common in the older patients with hypoglycemia.

Selected risk factors for hypoglycemia are discussed in more detail later.

Glucose Lowering Medications

Among the commonest risk factors for hypoglycemia in patients treated for DM is the use of glucose lowering agents that are not regulated by the ambient glucose concentration. These agents include all formulations of insulin and the sulfonylureas. The short-acting insulin secretagogues (repaglinide, nateglinide) are used less frequently but also pose hypoglycemia risk. Metformin is foundational therapy in most DM guidelines. It is not associated with increased hypoglycemia risk. Glucagonlike peptide-1 (GLP-1) receptor agonists and dipeptidyl peptidase-4 (DPP4) inhibitors lower glucose levels in glucose-dependent fashion and are not associated with hypoglycemia risk. Carbohydrase inhibitors and sodium-glucose cotransporter 2 (SGLT2) inhibitors work by different mechanisms of action, but both essentially have their greatest effect on prandial glycemic excursion and thus pose little risk of hypoglycemia. However, glucose lowering agents that are not associated with hypoglycemia when used as monotherapy or in combination may be associated with increased risk for hypoglycemia when used in conjunction with insulin or sulfonylureas.

In general, insulin therapy may still be necessary for adequate glycemic control in many patients. With increased availability of a wider range of glucose lowering agents, sulfonylurea use is declining, but the information on the impact on management of older patients is limited.

Other Medical Conditions that Are Associated with Hypoglycemia

Other medical conditions contribute to the increased risk for hypoglycemia. These conditions include decreased renal function, impaired liver function, certain classes of medication (especially with polypharmacy), and sarcopenia. Each of these is discussed in turn.

Renal compromise is often associated with increased risk for hypoglycemia, especially in patients treated with insulin or sulfonylureas.[26] Not only is the kidney important in the metabolism of insulin and some sulfonylureas but the kidney contributes to glucose counter-regulation if there is hypoglycemia. Because older patients often have diminished muscle mass, serum creatinine levels do not reflect renal function as well as in younger patients. However, laboratories now report an estimated glomerular filtration rate if they have the requisite information to make the calculation. These data include age, gender, race, and body weight. Because DM is associated with accelerated decline in renal function and because duration of disease is associated with increased need for insulin to achieve glycemic control, this combination of risk factors increases the risk for hypoglycemia in older patients.

Impaired liver function may contribute to the risk for hypoglycemia because the liver plays a key role in glucose counter-regulation via glycogenolysis and gluconeogenesis. Liver enzyme abnormalities and other markers of liver dysfunction are generally comparable in older patients. With increasing incidence of obesity and the associated nonalcoholic fatty liver disease, there is a corresponding increase in the risk for nonalcoholic steatohepatitis, which may in turn progress to cirrhosis. Once again liver disease risk is a function of age and duration of DM, so there may be some nominal increase in risk in older patients.

Polypharmacy increases the risk for hypoglycemia, likely because of medications that may be commonly used in older patients and also because cognitive decline in older patients means that confusion about proper medication administration may occur. Some medications increase the risk for hypoglycemia because they interfere with the patient's ability to detect the adrenergic/autonomic response. The most common class of medications is the β-blockers.[26] Angiotensin-converting enzyme inhibitors (ACEi) have also been associated with an increased risk for hypoglycemia.[26,40] ACEi are widely prescribed for their antihypertensive and renal protective effects. Even though ACEi hypoglycemia risk may be low in the context of declining renal function and polypharmacy, clinicians need to be aware of the risk. Ethanol ingestion is also associated with hypoglycemia risk, both because of the potential for impaired cognition and because ethanol impairs the gluconeogenic response to hypoglycemia.[41]

Sarcopenia is a complex process for which multiple mechanisms have been proposed, including insulin resistance, inflammation, and mitochondrial dysfunction.[13–15] Some understanding of basic physiology related to recovery from hypoglycemia and how the recovery from hypoglycemia may be impaired in patients with sarcopenia deserves brief discussion. Sarcopenia often accompanies the aging process and may contribute to hypoglycemia risk beyond its association with frailty. Muscle is a repository for stored glycogen, which in turn is an important substrate for glycogenolysis. Muscle is also a source of branched chain amino acids, a substrate for gluconeogenesis. Muscle wasting may be associated with increased risk for hypoglycemia.

Cardiovascular Disease

The role of hypoglycemia in CVD risk has been the source of much investigation.[20,28,29,36,42–49] The following are confounders in these analyses. Hypoglycemia is more likely to occur with increasing duration of DM and duration of disease is also associated with CVD. Glycemic variability is associated with increased risk of CVD and the risk for hypoglycemia.[49] In the Veterans Affairs Diabetes Trial, there was an association of severe hypoglycemia with CVD risk.[43] Importantly, the investigators noted: "The association between severe hypoglycemia and cardiovascular events increased significantly as overall cardiovascular risk increased." Yakubovich and Gerstein[47] analyzed clinical trials with several different designs and epidemiologic data to try to answer 3 key questions related to hypoglycemia and CVD in patents with DM: does an intervention that increases the risk of hypoglycemic episode increase the risk of serious cardiovascular outcomes? Are hypoglycemic episodes a risk factor for serious cardiovascular outcomes? Do hypoglycemic episodes precipitate serious cardiovascular events? In their conclusions, they note that "people who are prone to hypoglycemia are likely to be prone to other serious health outcomes due to the coexistence of other risk factors for these outcomes." They also acknowledge the need for further research.

Since the Yakubovich and Gerstein[47] publication, several large cardiovascular outcomes trials have shown the beneficial effects of selected classes of medications, most notably the SGLT2 inhibitors and some of the GLP-1 receptor agonists (see chapters Zehra Tekin and Robert S. Zimmerman's article, "Non-insulin Diabetes Therapies in Older Adults," in this issue and Adi Mehta and colleagues' article, "Diabetes and Heart Failure: A Marriage of Inconvenience," in this issue). Although hypoglycemia rates are low in these studies, whether hypoglycemia plays a role in CVD was not always evaluated. In a post hoc analysis of the Liraglutide Effect and Action in Diabetes: Evaluation of Cardiovascular Outcome Results (LEADER) trial, in which liraglutide was compared with a placebo, severe hypoglycemia was associated with increased cardiovascular events and all-cause mortality, but the cohort of patients with severe hypoglycemia was characterized by longer duration of DM, more insulin use, and renal disease.[46] The results of 2 trials in which the interventions had different rates of hypoglycemia but no differences in cardiovascular outcomes deserve comment. Trial Comparing Cardiovascular Safety of Insulin Degludec versus Insulin Glargine in Patients with Type 2 Diabetes at High Risk of Cardiovascular Events (DEVOTE).[50] There was no difference in cardiovascular events between the two regimens even though there were fewer hypoglycemia events with insulin degludec compared with insulin glargine. In a large randomized controlled trial of the DPP4 inhibitor, linagliptin, versus the sulfonylurea, glimepiride, there was no difference in CVD events even though there was increased hypoglycemia risk with the glimepiride compared with linagliptin.[51] At present, the role of hypoglycemia as a direct contributor to CVD events in older patients has not been proved convincingly.

Although there is still uncertainty about the relationships of hypoglycemia and CVD events, it is worth noting that there are several effects of hypoglycemia on risks for CVD events, including blood coagulations abnormalities, inflammation, endothelial dysfunction, and sympathetic nervous system activation.[29] Electrocardiogram abnormalities have also been observed in studies of hypoglycemia.[36]

In addition, HF has been associated with hypoglycemia. As with CVD, patients at risk for HF also have multiple risk factors for hypoglycemia. Proximate associations of hypoglycemia with worsening HF are currently limited. In a detailed study of hypoglycemia associated with hospitalization, Merrill and colleagues[52] evaluated 13,424 patients of whom 2484 had HF. Although hypoglycemia was associated with all-cause mortality, in their fully adjusted models severe hypoglycemia was not different in patients with versus without HF.

Mitigation of Hypoglycemia in Older Patients with Diabetes Mellitus

Selection of glucose lowering medications and glucose monitoring

Mitigation of hypoglycemia begins with the selection of glucose lowering agents that do not have an intrinsic risk of potential hypoglycemia, including insulin, sulfonylureas, and the short-acting insulin secretagogues (**Box 2**). Options include other oral agents such as metformin, DPP4 inhibitors, SGLT2 inhibitors, thiazolidinediones, and oral semaglutide. Metformin is usually foundational therapy in patients with DM[4–6] and concerns over HF and fractures have constrained the use of thiazolidinediones in

---

Box 2
Approaches to mitigating hypoglycemic risk in older patients with diabetes mellitus

1. Consider use of glucose lowering agents associated with increase hypoglycemia risk
   a. Insulin
   b. Sulfonylureas
   c. Short-acting insulin secretagogues (repaglinide, nateglinide)

2. Avoid medications that impair detection of hypoglycemia
   a. β-Blockers
   b. Psychotropic agents that may impair cognition or cause drowsiness

3. Implementation of glucose self-monitoring
   a. Self-monitoring of blood glucose
   b. Continuous glucose monitoring (selected patients at very high risk)

4. Mitigating physical impairments
   a. Visual impairment
      i. Medication boxes
      ii. Insulin pens/prefilled syringes
      iii. Glucose meters with voice synthesizers
   b. Cognitive impairment
      i. Simplifying medication regimens
      ii. Education of caregivers of interface of impaired memory and hypoglycemia

5. General education
   a. Nutrition, including use of glucose for hypoglycemia
   b. Effects of ethanol on hypoglycemia
   c. Detection of autonomic and neuroglycopenic symptoms

---

the past decade. There are several injectable GLP-1 receptor agonists, with twice-daily, daily, and weekly formulations all being available.

If patients need insulin therapy to achieve adequate glycemic control, then self-monitoring of blood glucose by fingerstick is readily available and flash monitoring and continuous glucose monitoring technology is also widely available. Closed loop systems, in which insulin administration via pump is linked to a continuous glucose monitor, are not yet widely used in the elderly.

Physical Limitations in Older Patients and Mitigating Hypoglycemia

Visual impairment in the elderly is common and is more frequent in patients with DM. Cataract formation is more common in patients with DM. Both proliferative diabetic retinopathy and DM-related macular edema are associated with visual compromise. Accurate oral medication administration can be facilitated with prefilled medication boxes. Nearly all insulin formulations are available in pens, and doses can be calculated by counting the clicks. Glucose monitoring devices with voice reporting are also readily available. These strategies require proper instruction by health care professionals, ideally to both the patient and a local relative or caregiver. Patients should have a ready source of rapid-acting glucose (tablets or gel) available for acute hypoglycemia management and instructions for appropriate additional foods to eat following an acute event. For patients who have frequent and/or severe hypoglycemia, glucagon (injectable or nasal) should be available, although injectable formulations are rarely self-administered.

Beyond appropriate use of glucose lowering medications and corresponding glucose monitoring, the following are also considerations in patients at risk for hypoglycemia. β-Blockers and other agents that may mask the adrenergic response of hypoglycemia should be avoided or used with caution if they are indicated. Patients and caregivers should be educated about detection of neuroglycopenia, including changes in cognition, confusion, nocturnal headaches, or nightmares. In patients with hypoglycemic unawareness, in which neuroglycopenia may be the only clinical symptom or sign, such education is especially important. Because hypoglycemia risk is associated with missed meals, the need for regular eating must be emphasized. For patients who choose to nap, an alarm should be set to avoid any prolonged period between eating or the duration of daytime sleep may increase the risk for hypoglycemia.

SUMMARY AND FUTURE VISION

Hypoglycemia in older patients is associated with increased age; insulin/sulfonylurea use; and multiple comorbidities, including renal disease, heart disease, and impaired cognition. Mitigation of hypoglycemia risk can be accomplished by selection of appropriate glucose lowering medication and education about hypoglycemia detection, nutritional approaches, and need for glucose self-monitoring. This strategy involves a team approach of health care providers, caregivers, and the patient.

Future data from clinical trials and real-world evidence should refine the understanding of the relationships among glucose lowering, glucose lowering medications, benefits to DM-related complications, and risks of hypoglycemia. Information on the appropriate use of medications with favorable clinical outcomes and low hypoglycemia risk should also be forthcoming. The hope is that this information may reduce the "evil" associated with DM.[1]

DISCLOSURE

B.J. Hoogwerf is a former employee and a minor stockholder of Eli Lilly and Co.

REFERENCES

1. Tattersall R. The pissing evil: a comprehensive history of diabetes mellitus. Ayeshire (Scotland): Swan and Horne; 2017.
2. Segel SA, Paramore DS, Cryer PE. Hypoglycemia-associated autonomic failure in advanced type 2 diabetes. Diabetes 2002;51(3):724–33.
3. Seaquist ER, Anderson J, Childs B, et al. Hypoglycemia and diabetes: a report of a workgroup of the American Diabetes Association and the Endocrine Society. Diabetes Care 2013;36(5):1384–95.
4. American Diabetes Association. 12. Older adults: standards of medical care in diabetes-2019. Diabetes Care 2019;42(Suppl 1):S139–47.
5. American Diabetes Association. 9. Pharmacologic approaches to glycemic treatment: standards of medical care in diabetes-2019. Diabetes Care 2019;42(Suppl 1):S90–102.
6. Garber AJ, Abrahamson MJ, Barzilay JI, et al. Consensus statement by the American Association of Clinical Endocrinologists and American College of Endocrinology on the comprehensive type 2 diabetes management algorithm - 2018 executive summary. Endocr Pract 2018;24(1):91–120.
7. Davies MJ, D'Alessio DA, Fradkin J, et al. Management of hyperglycemia in type 2 diabetes, 2018. A consensus report by the American Diabetes Association (ADA) and the European Association for the Study of Diabetes (EASD). Diabetes Care 2018;41(12):2669–701.
8. Home P. Controversies for glucose control targets in type 2 diabetes: exposing the common ground. Diabetes Care 2019;42(9):1615–23.

9. Ismail-Beigi F, Moghissi E, Tiktin M, et al. Individualizing glycemic targets in type 2 diabetes mellitus: implications of recent clinical trials. Ann Intern Med 2011; 154(8):554–9.

10. Tseng CL, Soroka O, Maney M, et al. Assessing potential glycemic overtreatment in persons at hypoglycemic risk. JAMA Intern Med 2014;174(2):259–68.

11. Andrews MA, O'Malley PG. Diabetes overtreatment in elderly individuals: risky business in need of better management. JAMA 2014;311(22):2326–7.

12. Weiner JZ, Gopalan A, Mishra P, et al. Use and discontinuation of insulin treatment among adults aged 75-70 years with type 2 diabetes. JAMA Intern Med 2019;179(12):1633–41.

13. Umegaki H. Sarcopenia and frailty in older patients with diabetes mellitus. Geriatr Gerontol Int 2016;16(3):293–9.

14. Morley JE. Diabetes, sarcopenia, and frailty. Clin Geriatr Med 2008;24(3): 455–69, vi.

15. Morley JE, Malmstrom TK, Rodriguez-Manas L, et al. Frailty, sarcopenia and diabetes. J Am Med Dir Assoc 2014;15(12):853–9.

16. Chiba Y, Kimbara Y, Kodera R, et al. Risk factors associated with falls in elderly patients with type 2 diabetes. J Diabetes Complications 2015;29(7):898–902.

17. Rajpathak SN, Fu C, Brodovicz KG, et al. Sulfonylurea use and risk of hip fractures among elderly men and women with type 2 diabetes. Drugs Aging 2015; 32(4):321–7.

18. Meneilly GS, Cheung E, Tuokko H. Counterregulatory hormone responses to hypoglycemia in the elderly patient with diabetes. Diabetes 1994;43(3):403–10.

19. Bremer JP, Jauch-Chara K, Hallschmid M, et al. Hypoglycemia unawareness in older compared with middle-aged patients with type 2 diabetes. Diabetes Care 2009;32(8):1513–7.

20. Pathak RD, Schroeder EB, Seaquist ER, et al. Severe hypoglycemia requiring medical intervention in a large cohort of adults with diabetes receiving care in U.S. Integrated health care delivery systems: 2005-2011. Diabetes Care 2016; 39(3):363–70.

21. Miller ME, Bonds DE, Gerstein HC, et al. The effects of baseline characteristics, glycaemia treatment approach, and glycated haemoglobin concentration on the risk of severe hypoglycaemia: post hoc epidemiological analysis of the ACCORD study. BMJ 2010;340:b5444.

22. Fu H, Xie W, Curtis B, et al. Identifying factors associated with hypoglycemia-related hospitalizations among elderly patients with T2DM in the US: a novel approach using influential variable analysis. Curr Med Res Opin 2014;30(9): 1787–93.

23. Bramlage P, Gitt AK, Binz C, et al. Oral antidiabetic treatment in type-2 diabetes in the elderly: balancing the need for glucose control and the risk of hypoglycemia. Cardiovasc Diabetol 2012;11:122.

24. Akram K, Pedersen-Bjergaard U, Carstensen B, et al. Frequency and risk factors of severe hypoglycaemia in insulin-treated Type 2 diabetes: a cross-sectional survey. Diabet Med 2006;23(7):750–6.

25. Bordier L, Buysschaert M, Bauduceau B, et al. Predicting factors of hypoglycaemia in elderly type 2 diabetes patients: contributions of the GERODIAB study. Diabetes Metab 2015;41(4):301–3.

26. Chelliah A, Burge MR. Hypoglycaemia in elderly patients with diabetes mellitus: causes and strategies for prevention. Drugs Aging 2004;21(8):511–30.

27. Chin SO, Rhee SY, Chon S, et al. Hypoglycemia is associated with dementia in elderly patients with type 2 diabetes mellitus: an analysis based on the Korea National Diabetes Program Cohort. Diabetes Res Clin Pract 2016;122:54–61.
28. Chow E, Bernjak A, Williams S, et al. Risk of cardiac arrhythmias during hypoglycemia in patients with type 2 diabetes and cardiovascular risk. Diabetes 2014; 63(5):1738–47.
29. Connelly KA, Yan AT, Leiter LA, et al. Cardiovascular implications of hypoglycemia in diabetes mellitus. Circulation 2015;132(24):2345–50.
30. Corsonello A, Pedone C, Corica F, et al. Antihypertensive drug therapy and hypoglycemia in elderly diabetic patients treated with insulin and/or sulfonylureas. Gruppo Italiano di Farmacovigilanza nell'Anziano (GIFA). Eur J Epidemiol 1999; 15(10):893–901.
31. Fang F, Xiao H, Li C, et al. Fasting glucose level is associated with nocturnal hypoglycemia in elderly male patients with type 2 diabetes. Aging Male 2013;16(3): 132–6.
32. Fukuda M, Doi K, Sugawara M, et al. Survey of hypoglycemia in elderly people with type 2 diabetes mellitus in Japan. J Clin Med Res 2015;7(12):967–78.
33. Kagansky N, Levy S, Rimon E, et al. Hypoglycemia as a predictor of mortality in hospitalized elderly patients. Arch Intern Med 2003;163(15):1825–9.
34. Muratli S, Tufan F, Soyluk O, et al. Importance of hypoglycemia on the risk of Alzheimer's disease in elderly subjects with diabetes mellitus. Clin Interv Aging 2015;10:1789–91.
35. Pilotto A, Noale M, Maggi S, et al. Hypoglycemia is independently associated with multidimensional impairment in elderly diabetic patients. Biomed Res Int 2014;2014:906103.
36. Pistrosch F, Ganz X, Bornstein SR, et al. Risk of and risk factors for hypoglycemia and associated arrhythmias in patients with type 2 diabetes and cardiovascular disease: a cohort study under real-world conditions. Acta Diabetol 2015;52(5): 889–95.
37. Punthakee Z, Miller ME, Launer LJ, et al. Poor cognitive function and risk of severe hypoglycemia in type 2 diabetes: post hoc epidemiologic analysis of the ACCORD trial. Diabetes Care 2012;35(4):787–93.
38. Seaquist ER, Miller ME, Bonds DE, et al. The impact of frequent and unrecognized hypoglycemia on mortality in the ACCORD study. Diabetes Care 2012; 35(2):409–14.
39. Stepka M, Rogala H, Czyzyk A. Hypoglycemia: a major problem in the management of diabetes in the elderly. Aging (Milano) 1993;5(2):117–21.
40. Morris AD, Boyle DI, McMahon AD, et al. ACE inhibitor use is associated with hospitalization for severe hypoglycemia in patients with diabetes. DARTS/ MEMO Collaboration. Diabetes Audit and Research in Tayside, Scotland. Medicines Monitoring Unit. Diabetes Care 1997;20(9):1363–7.
41. Pedersen-Bjergaard U, Reubsaet JL, Nielsen SL, et al. Psychoactive drugs, alcohol, and severe hypoglycemia in insulin-treated diabetes: analysis of 141 cases. Am J Med 2005;118(3):307–10.
42. Cha SA, Yun JS, Lim TS, et al. Severe hypoglycemia and cardiovascular or all-cause mortality in patients with type 2 diabetes. Diabetes Metab J 2016;40(3): 202–10.
43. Davis SN, Duckworth W, Emanuele N, et al. Effects of severe hypoglycemia on cardiovascular outcomes and death in the veterans affairs diabetes trial. Diabetes Care 2019;42(1):157–63.

44. Lee AK, Warren B, Lee CJ, et al. The association of severe hypoglycemia with incident cardiovascular events and mortality in adults with type 2 diabetes. Diabetes Care 2018;41(1):104–11.
45. Snell-Bergeon JK, Wadwa RP. Hypoglycemia, diabetes, and cardiovascular disease. Diabetes Technol Ther 2012;14(Suppl 1):S51–8.
46. Zinman B, Marso SP, Christiansen E, et al. Hypoglycemia, cardiovascular outcomes, and death: the LEADER experience. Diabetes Care 2018;41(8):1783–91.
47. Yakubovich N, Gerstein HC. Serious cardiovascular outcomes in diabetes: the role of hypoglycemia. Circulation 2011;123(3):342–8.
48. Paty BW. The role of hypoglycemia in cardiovascular outcomes in diabetes. Can J Diabetes 2015;39(Suppl 5):S155–9.
49. Sun B, He F, Gao Y, et al. Prognostic impact of visit-to-visit glycemic variability on the risks of major adverse cardiovascular outcomes and hypoglycemia in patients with different glycemic control and type 2 diabetes. Endocrine 2019; 64(3):536–43.
50. Marso SP, McGuire DK, Zinman B, et al. Efficacy and safety of Degludec versus Glargine in Type 2 Diabetes. N Engl J Med 2017;377(8):723–32.
51. Rosenstock J, Kahn SE, Johansen OE, et al. Effect of linagliptin vs glimepiride on major adverse cardiovascular outcomes in patients with type 2 diabetes: the CAROLINA randomized clinical trial. JAMA 2019;322(12):1155–66.
52. Merrill JD, Dungan KM. Hypoglycaemia in hospitalized patients with or without heart failure. Diabetes Obes Metab 2018;20(10):2472–6.

Cognitive Dysfunction in Older Adults with Type 2 Diabetes

Links, Risks, and Clinical Implications

Alan Sinclair, MSc, MD, FRCP[a,b,]*, Ahmed Abdelhafiz, MD, FRCP[c]

KEYWORDS

- Older people • Diabetes mellitus • Cognitive dysfunction • Management

KEY POINTS

- As population ages, the prevalence of comorbid diabetes and cognitive dysfunction increases.
- The development of cognitive dysfunction will have significant consequences on the care for older people with diabetes.
- Health care professionals and health care systems should develop policies that ensure delivering of a holistic care plans that focus on quality of life of these patients with complex needs.

INTRODUCTION

The global prevalence of diabetes mellitus was 8.4% of the total population in 2017 and is expected to reach approximately 10% in 2045.[1] The lifetime risk of developing diabetes is 22.4% for women and 18.9% for men from the age of 60 years onward.[1] The rise in the prevalence of diabetes is likely to be due to the increase in life expectancy and the associated increased risk of developing diabetes with increasing age. Almost half (44%) of the population with diabetes is older than 65 years, with a prevalence of diabetes that peaks (22%) at 75 to 79 years of age.[1] In old age, diabetes is associated with high comorbidity burden and increased prevalence of geriatric syndromes, including cognitive dysfunction. Cognitive dysfunction commonly coexists with diabetes and proportionally increases with increasing age. In the United States, approximately 16% of people aged ≥65 years and 24% of those aged ≥75 years with diabetes have dementia.[2] In France, the estimated prevalence of cognitive

[a] Foundation for Diabetes Research in Older People, Diabetes Frail Ltd, Droitwich Spa WR9 0QH, UK; [b] Kings College, London SE1 9NH, UK; [c] Department of Geriatric Medicine, Rotherham General Hospital, Moorgate Road, Rotherham S60 2UD, UK
* Corresponding author.
E-mail address: Sinclair.5@btinternet.com

Clin Geriatr Med 36 (2020) 407–417
https://doi.org/10.1016/j.cger.2020.04.002
0749-0690/20/© 2020 Elsevier Inc. All rights reserved.

geriatric.theclinics.com

impairment among older people (aged 75–79 years) with diabetes is approximately 29%.[3] In an audit of 11 nursing homes in the United Kingdom, 56% of older people with diabetes (mean age 80.6 years) were found to have some form of dementia.[4] Risk factors that lead to cognitive dysfunction in older people with diabetes may include shared factors that predispose to diabetes, such as obesity and insulin resistance, diabetes-related factors such as chronic low-grade inflammation and hyperglycemia or hypoglycemia, and diabetes-associated factors such as cardiovascular complications.[5,6] Diabetes mellitus is associated with varying degrees of cognitive dysfunction that ranges from cognitive decline and mild cognitive impairment (MCI) to dementia (**Table 1**).[7–9] With increasing aging of the population, the prevalence of comorbid diabetes and dementia is likely to increase. Cognitive dysfunction, especially in the executive domains, may interfere with diabetes self-care management and may lead to a poor glycemic control. Also, with the progression of dementia and the development behavioral abnormalities, diabetes management will represent a unique challenge for health care professionals. Therefore, early recognition of the presence of dementia in an older patient with diabetes may lead to a better outcome. Individually tailored strategies that accommodate and adjust to the patients' cognitive abilities to optimize their capacity for self-care will be required for older people with comorbid diabetes and dementia. This article reviews the association and the impact of cognitive dysfunction on older people with diabetes and explores the management challenges in this group of complex patients.

Table 1
Stages of cognitive dysfunction in older people with diabetes[59]

Parameter	Stage 1 Cognitive Decline	Stage 2 Mild Cognitive Impairment	Stage 3 Dementia
Cognitive changes	Subtle cognitive changes in ≥ 1 domains	Clear cognitive changes in ≥ 1 domains	Obvious cognitive changes in multiple domains
Age group	Affect all ages	Mostly patients >60 y	Primarily patients >60 y
Clinical picture	Apparently normal cognition, only detectable on neuropsychological assessment.	Cognitive testing shows deficits that do not meet the criteria for dementia diagnosis and involve only subtle impairment in activities of daily living.	Decline in executive function, such as reasoning, planning and problem-solving
Effect on self-care	No effect on self-care for those on oral therapy, but difficulties with complex insulin regimen.	Affect self-care management.	Grossly affect self-care, inability to understand or remember instructions
Course	Slow progression	May regress to normal cognition, remain stable or progress to dementia.	Progressive course

DIABETES AND DEMENTIA: THE LINK

Diabetes and dementia may share a common pathogenic link. In Alzheimer disease (AD), increased cerebral insulin resistance appears to be the central feature of this metabolic-cognitive syndrome, suggesting that AD is an insulin-resistant brain state or type 3 diabetes.[10] The increased cerebral insulin resistance is due to impaired insulin signaling.[10] Adequate insulin signaling is responsible for the regulation of acetylcholine production, learning, and memory, therefore, impairment of insulin signaling is associated with accelerated neuronal dysfunction and cognitive decline.[11] The link between diabetes mellitus and AD is also manifested by the accumulation of amyloid protein in the β-cells of the pancreas and in the brain. Both diabetes mellitus and AD are protein misfolding disorders that lead to the formation and accumulation of proteinaceous misfolded aggregates: the islet amyloid polypeptide in the pancreas in case of diabetes and the amyloid-beta (Aβ) and tau in the brain in case of AD, which may interact by cross-seeding that links both diseases with a common pathogenic mechanism.[12] Increased oxidative stress and increased production of advanced glycation end products are other shared pathogenic factors that lead to impaired cellular functions.[13] Another link is the low level of the brain-derived neurotropic factor, a growth factor that promotes brain function and has antidiabetes effects, in persons with comorbid diabetes and dementia.[14] Vascular dementia may be linked to diabetes through diabetes-related macro and micro cerebrovascular diseases, chronic inflammation, and endothelial dysfunction.[5] Other diabetes-associated comorbidities, such as obesity and hypertension, may be contributing cardiovascular risk factors. However, it has been shown that the association between diabetes mellitus and dementia is only partially mediated through cerebrovascular disease, suggesting that diabetes mellitus may have a direct effect on brain function independent of cerebrovascular disease and is the main driver of the dementia risk.[15,16] Genetic factors such as the APOE ε4 allele increases the risk of atherosclerosis and is associated with increased risk for cerebral amyloid angiopathy and cognitive decline.[17] Nutritional factors such as low intakes of carotene, vitamin B2, pantothenate, calcium, and green vegetables (suggesting malnutrition) and poor oral health (suggesting chronic inflammation) have been shown to be associated with cognitive decline in older people with diabetes.[18,19] The blood-brain barrier (BBB) maintains homeostasis in the central nervous system by regulating ion balance, facilitating nutritional transport, and preventing influx of potentially neurotoxic molecules from the circulation, and it has been shown that increased BBB permeability is another link increasing the risk of both diabetes and dementia.[20] High and low blood glucose levels are other pathogenic factors for dementia. It has been demonstrated that high blood glucose level is a risk factor for dementia regardless of the diabetes status or cardiovascular risk factors, suggesting that glucotoxicity may have a direct deleterious effect on the aging brain.[21,22] On the other hand, repeated episodes of low blood glucose level or hypoglycemia may also induce brain cell damage that leads to cognitive dysfunction in a graded relationship[23] (**Fig. 1**).

DIABETES AND DEMENTIA: THE RISK

Diabetes increases the risk of cognitive dysfunction. Previous and recent meta-analyses have demonstrated that diabetes increased the risk of all types of dementia by almost twofold.[24–31] Type 1 diabetes also increases the risk of dementia by almost 80% in those older than 60 years.[32] The presence of diabetes at a younger age appears to increase the risk of dementia in later life.[33,34] Diabetes also increases

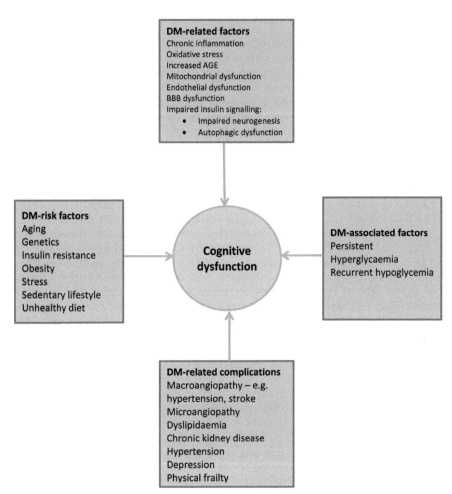

DM-related factors
Chronic inflammation
Oxidative stress
Increased AGE
Mitochondrial dysfunction
Endothelial dysfunction
BBB dysfunction
Impaired insulin signalling:
- Impaired neurogenesis
- Autophagic dysfunction

DM-risk factors
Aging
Genetics
Insulin resistance
Obesity
Stress
Sedentary lifestyle
Unhealthy diet

Cognitive dysfunction

DM-associated factors
Persistent Hyperglycaemia
Recurrent hypoglycemia

DM-related complications
Macroangiopathy – e.g. hypertension, stroke
Microangiopathy
Dyslipidaemia
Chronic kidney disease
Hypertension
Depression
Physical frailty

Fig. 1. The pathogenic link between diabetes mellitus and cognitive dysfunction. AGE, advanced glycation end products; BBB, blood-brain barrier; DM, diabetes mellitus.

the risk of MCI as well as its progression to dementia, which was accelerated in the presence of other cardiovascular risk factors or metabolic syndrome.[27,28,31,35] In the Atherosclerosis Risk in Communities Study, poor glycemic control (HbA1c ≥53 mmol/mol, 7.0%) or longer duration of diabetes (>9 years) had a larger cognitive decline compared with better glycemic control (HbA1c <53 mmol/mol, 7.0%) or shorter duration (<3 years) of diabetes ($P = .07$ and <0.001, respectively).[36] Also, cognitive decline was significantly higher in persons with prediabetes, defined as HbA1c 38.8 to 46.4 mmol/mol (5.7%–6.4%), than those without a diagnosis of diabetes or had an HbA1c <38.8 mmol/mol (5.7%).[35] Both high and low blood glucose levels appear to increase the risk of dementia. In older people (mean age 76 years), higher blood glucose levels (6.4 vs 5.5 mmol/L) (115 vs 100 mg/dL), even without a diagnosis of diabetes, have been shown to be associated with an increased risk of dementia (hazard ratio [HR] 1.18, 95% confidence interval [CI] 1.04–1.33, $P = .01$).[21] On the other hand, low blood glucose or hypoglycemia is a risk factor for cognitive dysfunction, as glucose is the main source of cerebral energy.[37–42] Although transient hypoglycemia may lead to reversible impairment of cognitive function, persistent or severe hypoglycemia may result in a permanent neuronal damage.[43] The risk of dementia increases proportionally with increasing frequency of hypoglycemic episodes. It has been shown that the risk of dementia increases by 26% for 1 episode of hypoglycemia, 80% for 2 episodes, and 94% for 3 or more episodes.[44] The dose-response relationship between the frequency of severe hypoglycemia and incidence of dementia has also been shown in other studies.[23] Recently, hypoglycemia has been shown to be associated with cognitive decline, low brain volume, and dementia.[42] Low blood glucose (<4.7 mmol/L) (<85 mg/dL) also increased the risk of MCI in older people without history of diabetes (relative risk 1.57, 95% CI 1.14–2.32), suggesting a deleterious effect of low glucose on normal brains.[45] The relationship between hypoglycemia and dementia has also been shown in older people newly diagnosed with diabetes mellitus.[38] Three studies have shown a relationship between hypoglycemia and increased risk of neurocognitive dysfunction and MCI.[46–48] Hypoglycemia was associated with cognitive decline in care home residents.[41] Recent meta-analyses investigating the risk of cognitive dysfunction in older people with diabetes are summarized in **Table 2**, and recent studies exploring the relationship between hypoglycemia and cognitive dysfunction are summarized in **Table 3** (see the Byron J. Hoogwerf's article, "Hypoglycemia in the Older Patient," elsewhere in this issue, for additional discussion.)

DIABETES AND DEMENTIA: CLINICAL IMPLICATIONS

Diabetes mellitus is a chronic condition that requires good cognitive function to execute self-care tasks, to achieve good glycemic control, and to avoid acute and long-term diabetes-related complications. With memory and executive function impairments associated with dementia, older people with comorbid diabetes and dementia will be less compliant with the prescribed regimens, have an erratic eating pattern, and are at risk of weight loss and malnutrition. In a cross-sectional study of 1398 persons with diabetes aged ≥60 years, cognitive dysfunction was associated with significant difficulty in adherence to diet and exercise.[49] Impairment in executive function, memory, and global cognition have been shown to be significantly correlated with impairment in diabetes-specific numeracy ability, diabetes knowledge, insulin dose adjustment, insulin injection skills, medications adherence, self-care activity, and glucose monitoring, which were all exacerbated by increasing age.[50] Comorbid diabetes and dementia increases the risk of hypoglycemia. It has been shown that older people with comorbid diabetes and dementia have threefold the risk of hypoglycemia compared with those with diabetes alone (14.2% vs 6.3%, $P<.001$, adjusted HR 3.1, 95% CI 1.5–6.6).[51] The risk of hypoglycemia increases proportionally with the severity of dementia.[52,53] Dementia in older people with diabetes also increases the risk of frailty. Dementia appears to be linked to frailty, and both may share a common pathogenic pathway that includes increased oxidative stress, impaired repair, and unhealthy life style.[54,55] Dementia associated with diabetes-related metabolic abnormalities has been shown to be associated with frailty more often than diabetes-associated AD, and this is likely to be due to increased inflammatory processes and oxidative stress in these patients.[56,57] The new term "cognitive frailty" has been recently introduced by an international consensus group to describe the simultaneous presence of cognitive impairment and physical frailty, highlighting the link between both conditions.[58] Many tasks in activities of daily living will require intact physical and cognitive functions and the development of cognitive frailty will further lead to a negative impact on self-care of older people with diabetes.

Table 2
Recent meta-analyses investigating the risk of cognitive dysfunction in older people with diabetes

Meta-Analysis	Patients	Aim to	Main Findings
Ninomiya,[26] 2014, 18 studies	Total 55,651 subjects, average age 69–88 y, F/U 2.1–15 y.	Examine risk of dementia in people with diabetes.	Diabetes was associated with increased risk of A. All dementia (HR 1.7, 95% CI 1.5–1.8). B. AD (1.6, 1.4–1.8). C. VD (2.2, 1.7–2.8).
Cooper et al,[27] 2015, 7 studies	Total 12,283 subjects, age ≥55 y.	Predict progression of MCI to dementia.	Diabetes was a risk factor for progression from MCI to dementia (OR 1.65, 95% CI 1.12–2.43).
Li et al,[28] 2016, 60 studies	Total 14,821 participants, age NR.	Identify risk factors for progression from MCI to AD.	Diabetes increased risk of progression from MCI to AD (RR 1.52, 95% CI 1.2–1.91).
Chatterjee et al,[29] 2016, 14 studies	Total 2,310,330 subjects, aged average 43–83 y.	Estimate gender-specific diabetes-associated risk of dementia.	Diabetes increased risk of A. VD (OR 2.34, 95% CI 1.86–2.94 in women and 1.73, 1.61–1.85 in men). B. Non-VD (1.53, 1.35–1.73 in women and 1.49, 1.31–1.69 in men).
Zhang et al,[30] 2017, 17 studies	Total 1,746,777 subjects of whom 710,858 had diabetes.	Examine association of diabetes with AD.	A. Diabetes increased risk of AD (RR 1.53, 95% CI 1.42–1.63). B. Risk was higher in Eastern (1.62, 1.49–1.75) compared with Western (1.36, 1.18–1.53) populations.
Kingshuk et al,[31] 2018, 12 studies	Total 6865 participants, age NR.	Quantify RR of progression from MCI to dementia.	Participants with diabetes and MCI had increased risk of progression to dementia (OR 1.53, 95% CI 1.20–1.97) compared with those with MCI but no diabetes.

Abbreviations: AD, Alzheimer disease; CI, confidence interval; F/U, follow-up; HR, hazard ratio; MCI, mild cognitive impairment; NR, not reported; OR, odds ratio; RR, relative risk; VD, vascular dementia.

Table 3
Recent studies exploring the effect of hypoglycemia on the risk of cognitive dysfunction in older people with diabetes

Study	Patients	Aim to	Main Findings
Feinkohl et al,[37] prospective, UK, 2014 UK	831 patients with DM age 60–75 y, F/U 4 y.	Investigate association of hypoglycemia and cognitive decline, a standardized general ability factor g was used.	A. Incident hypoglycemia was associated with poorer cognitive ability at baseline (OR for lowest tertile of g 2.04; 95% CI 1.25–3.31, P = .004). B. Both history of hypoglycemia and incident hypoglycemia were associated with greater cognitive decline during follow-up (mean adjusted follow-up gs were −0.23 vs 0.03 [P = .04] and −0.21 vs 0.05 [P = .03], respectively).
Haroon et al,[38] prospective, Canada, 2015	89,115 patients, median age 73Y, F/U 5 y.	Determine risk of dementia in patients with or without DM.	Hypoglycemia predicted dementia (HR 1.73, 95% CI 1.62–1.84).
Chin et al,[39] prospective, Korea, 2016	1957 patients with DM, aged ≥60 y, F/U 3.4 y.	Investigate association of hypoglycaemia with dementia or cognitive dysfunction.	A. Hypoglycemia was independently associated with dementia (HR 2.69, 95% CI 1.08–6.69, P = .03). B. There was a significant linear trend between dementia and number of hypoglycemic events (P = .03).
Mehta et al,[40] retrospective, UK, 2017	53,055 patients >65 y with DM.	Evaluate association of hypoglycemia and dementia.	A. Hypoglycemia increased risk of dementia (HR 1.27, 95% CI 1.06–1.51). B. Risk of dementia increased with increasing number of hypoglycemic episodes: 1 episode (HR 1.26, 95% CI 1.03–1.54), 2 episodes (1.5, 1.09–2.08).

(continued on next page)

Table 3
(continued)

Study	Patients	Aim to	Main Findings
Alonso et al,[41] cross-sectional, Spain, 2018	654 care home residents, mean age 82.4 y.	Establish relation of hypoglycemia and cognitive impairment.	In residents with DM, low HbA1c (<6.0%) was associated with higher cognitive impairment ($P = .04$).
Lee et al,[42] cross-sectional prospective, US, 2018	2001 patients with DM, mean age 76 y, F/U 15 y.	Evaluate association of hypoglycemia with cognitive decline, brain volume, and dementia.	Severe hypoglycemia was associated with A. Dementia (OR 2.34, 95% CI 1.04–5.27). B. Small brain volume, (−0.308 SD, −0.612 to −0.004). C. 15 y cognitive change (−0.14 SD, −0.34–0.06). D. Incident dementia (HR 2.54, 95% CI 1.78–3.63).

Abbreviations: CI, confidence interval; DM, diabetes mellitus; F/U, follow-up; HR, hazard ratio; OR, odds ratio; SD, standard deviation.

SUMMARY

Cognitive dysfunction is an important complication in older people with diabetes, and both index conditions may share a common pathogenic pathway. We also recognize that the global prevalence of comorbid diabetes and dementia is increasing, which poses important personal and public health issues. With the progression of dementia and the development of behavioral abnormalities, diabetes management will continue to represent a unique challenge for health care professionals.

Future research requires clinical trials to address issues relating to glycemic control, medication management, and diabetes-related self-care in older people with comorbid diabetes and dementia. Research into system-wide issues that include access of this group of patients to regular assessments, barriers of achieving individualized care plans, appropriate management, overall care, and the applicability of different approaches and interventions in different settings is also required.

DISCLOSURE

The authors have nothing to disclose.

REFERENCES

1. Cho NH, Shaw JE, Karuranga S, et al. IDF Diabetes Atlas: global estimates of diabetes prevalence for 2017 and projections for 2045. Diabetes Res Clin Pract 2018;138:271–81.

2. Thorpe CT, Thorpe JM, Kind AJ, et al. Receipt of monitoring of diabetes mellitus in older adults with comorbid dementia. J Am Geriatr Soc 2012;60:644–51.

3. Bordier L, Doucet J, Boudet J, et al. Update on cognitive decline and dementia in elderly patients with diabetes. Diabetes Metab 2014;40:331–7.

4. Gadsby R, Barker P, Sinclair A. People living with diabetes resident in nursing homes–assessing levels of disability and nursing needs. Diabet Med 2011;28: 778–80.
5. Middleton LE, affe K. Promising strategies for the prevention of dementia. Arch Neurol 2009;66:1210–5.
6. Kalyani RR, Corriere M, Ferrucci L. Age-related and disease-related muscle loss: the effect of diabetes, obesity, and other diseases. Lancet Diabetes Endocrinol 2014;10:819–29.
7. Arvanitakis Z, Wilson RS, Bienias JL, et al. Diabetes mellitus and risk of Alzheimer disease and decline in cognitive function. Arch Neurol 2004;61:661–6.
8. Luchsinger JA, Reitz C, Patel B, et al. Relation of diabetes to mild cognitive impairment. Arch Neurol 2007;64:570–5.
9. Ahtiluoto S, Polvikoski T, Peltonen M, et al. Diabetes, Alzheimer disease and vascular dementia: a population-based neuropathologic study. Neurology 2011;75:1195–202.
10. Frisardi V, Solfrizzi V, Capurso C, et al. Is insulin resistant brain state a central feature of the metabolic cognitive syndrome? J Alzheimers Dis 2010;21:57–63.
11. de la Monte SM. Insulin resistance and Alzheimer's disease. BMB Rep 2009;42: 475–81.
12. Moreno-Gonzalez I, Edwards G III, Salvadores N, et al. Molecular interaction between type 2 diabetes and Alzheimer's disease through cross-seeding of protein misfolding. Mol Psychiatry 2017;22:1327–34.
13. Akter K, Lanza EA, Martin SA, et al. Diabetes mellitus and Alzheimer's disease: shared pathology and treatment? Br J Clin Pharmacol 2011;71:365–76.
14. Passaro A, Nora ED, Morieri ML, et al. Brain-derived neurotrophic factor plasma levels: relationship with dementia and diabetes in the elderly population. J Gerontol A Biol Sci Med Sci 2015;70:294–302.
15. Lu ZK, Li M, Yuan J, et al. The role of cerebrovascular disease and the association between diabetes mellitus and dementia among aged Medicare beneficiaries. Int J Geriatr Psychiatry 2016;31:92–8.
16. Bangen KJ, Gu Y, Gross AL, et al. Relationship between type 2 diabetes mellitus and cognitive change in a multi-ethnic elderly cohort. J Am Geriatr Soc 2015;63: 1075–83.
17. Takeda M, Martinez R, Kudo T, et al. Apolipoprotein E and central nervous system disorders: reviews of clinical findings. Psychiatry Clin Neurosci 2010;64:592–607.
18. Araki A, Yoshimura Y, Sakurai T, et al. Low intakes of carotene, vitamin B2, pantothenate and calcium predict cognitive decline among elderly patients with diabetes mellitus: the Japanese Elderly Diabetes Intervention Trial. Geriatr Gerontol Int 2017;17:1168–75.
19. Batty GD, Li Q, Huxley R, et al. Oral disease in relation to future risk of dementia and cognitive decline: prospective cohort study based on the Action in Diabetes and Vascular Disease: preterax and Diamicron Modified-Release Controlled Evaluation (ADVANCE) trial. Eur Psychiatry 2013;28:49–52.
20. Janelidze S, Hertze J, Nägga K, et al. Increased blood-brain barrier permeability is associated with dementia and diabetes but not amyloid pathology or APOE genotype. Neurobiol Aging 2017;51:104–12.
21. Crane PK, Walker R, Hubbard RA, et al. Glucose levels and risk of dementia. N Engl J Med 2013;369:540–8.
22. Kerti L, Witte AV, Winkler A, et al. Higher glucose levels associated with lower memory and reduced hippocampal microstructure. Neurology 2013;81:1746–52.

23. Lin CH, Sheu WHH. Hypoglycaemic episodes and risk of dementia in diabetes mellitus: 7-year follow-up study. J Intern Med 2013;273:102–10.

24. Cheng G, Huang C, Deng H, et al. Diabetes as a risk factor for dementia and mild cognitive impairment: a meta-analysis of longitudinal studies. Intern Med J 2012; 42:484–91.

25. Gudala K, Bansal D, Schifano F, et al. Diabetes mellitus and risk of dementia: a meta-analysis of prospective observational studies. J Diabetes Investig 2013;4:640–50.

26. Ninomiya T. Diabetes mellitus and dementia. Curr Diab Rep 2014;14:487.

27. Cooper C, Sommerlad A, Lyketsos CG, et al. Modifiable predictors of dementia in mild cognitive impairment: a systematic review and meta-analysis. Am J Psychiatry 2015;172:323–34.

28. Li JQ, Tan L, Wang HF, et al. Risk factors for predicting progression from mild cognitive impairment to Alzheimer's disease: a systematic review and meta-analysis of cohort studies. J Neurol Neurosurg Psychiatry 2016;87:476–84.

29. Chatterjee S, Peters SA, Woodward M, et al. Type 2 diabetes as a risk factor for dementia in women compared with men: a pooled analysis of 2.3 million people comprising more than 100,000 cases of dementia. Diabetes Care 2016;39:300–7.

30. Zhang J, Chen C, Hua S, et al. An updated meta-analysis of cohort studies: diabetes and risk of Alzheimer's disease. Diabetes Res Clin Pract 2017;124:41–7.

31. Kingshuk P, Mukadam N, Petersen I, et al. Mild cognitive impairment and progression to dementia in people with diabetes, prediabetes and metabolic syndrome: a systematic review and meta-analysis. Soc Psychiatry Psychiatr Epidemiol 2018;53:1149–60.

32. Whitmer RA, Biessels GJ, Quesenberry CP, et al. Type 1 diabetes and risk of dementia in late life: the Kaiser diabetes & cognitive aging study. Alzheimers Dement 2015;11(Suppl):179–80.

33. Davis WA, Zilkens RR, Starkstein SE, et al. Dementia onset, incidence and risk in type 2 diabetes: a matched cohort study with the Fremantle Diabetes Study Phase I. Diabetologia 2017;60:89–97.

34. Meng XF, Yu JT, Wang HF, et al. Midlife vascular risk factors and the risk of Alzheimer's disease: a systematic review and meta-analysis. J Alzheimers Dis 2014; 42:1295–310.

35. Roberts RO, Knopman DS, Geda YE, et al. Association of diabetes with amnestic and non-amnestic mild cognitive impairment. Alzheimers Dement 2014;10:18–26.

36. Rawlings AM, Sharrett AR, Schneider ALC, et al. Diabetes in midlife and cognitive change over 20 years: the atherosclerosis risk in communities neurocognitive study. Ann Intern Med 2014;161:785–93.

37. Feinkohl I, Aung PP, Keller M, et al. Severe hypoglycemia and cognitive decline in older people with type 2 diabetes: the Edinburgh type 2 diabetes study. Diabetes Care 2014;37:507–15.

38. Haroon NN, Austin PC, Shah BR, et al. Risk of dementia in seniors with newly diagnosed diabetes: a population-based study. Diabetes Care 2015;38:1868–75.

39. Chin SO, Rhee SY, Chon S, et al. Hypoglycemia is associated with dementia in elderly patients with type 2 diabetes mellitus: an analysis based on the Korea National Diabetes Program Cohort. Diabetes Res Clin Pract 2016;122:54–61.

40. Mehta HB, Mehta V, Goodwin JS. Association of hypoglycemia with subsequent dementia in older patients with type 2 diabetes mellitus. Gerontol A Biol Sci Med Sci 2017;72:1110–6.

41. Alonso MAC, Santos JMM, Vilanova MI, et al. Over effective control of glycemic levels could cause cognitive decline in diabetic geriatric population. Neurol Neurosci Res 2017;1:3.

42. Lee AK, Rawlings AM, Lee CJ, et al. Severe hypoglycaemia, mild cognitive impairment, dementia and brain volumes in older adults with type 2 diabetes: the Atherosclerosis Risk in Communities (ARIC) cohort study. Diabetologia 2018;61:1956–65.
43. Bree AJ, Puente EC, Daphna-Iken D, et al. Diabetes increases brain damage caused by severe hypoglycemia. Am J Physiol Endocrinol Metab 2009;297: E194–201.
44. Whitmer RA, Karter AJ, Yaffe K, et al. Hypoglycemic episodes and risk of dementia in older patients with type 2 diabetes mellitus. JAMA 2009;301:1565–72.
45. Wang F, Zhao M, Han Z, et al. Long-term subclinical hyperglycemia and hypoglycemia as independent risk factors for mild cognitive impairment in elderly people. Tohoku J Exp Med 2017;242:121–8.
46. Duning T, van den Heuvel I, Dickmann A, et al. Hypoglycemia aggravates critical illness-induced neurocognitive dysfunction. Diabetes Care 2010;33:639–44.
47. Aung PP, Strachan MW, Frier BM, et al. Severe hypoglycaemia and late-life cognitive ability in older people with type 2 diabetes: the Edinburgh type 2 diabetes study. Diabet Med 2012;29:328–36.
48. Gao Y, Xiao Y, Miao R, et al. The characteristic of cognitive function in Type 2 diabetes mellitus. Diabetes Res Clin Pract 2015;109:299–305.
49. Feil DG, Zhu CW, Sultzer DL. The relationship between cognitive impairment and diabetes self-management in a population-based community sample of older adults with Type 2 diabetes. J Behav Med 2012;35:190–9.
50. Tomlin A, Sinclair A. The influence of cognition on self-management of type 2 diabetes in older people. Psychol Res Behav Manag 2016;9:7–20.
51. Yaffe K, Falvey CM, Hamilton N, et al, for the Health ABC Study. Association between hypoglycemia and dementia in a biracial cohort of older adults with diabetes mellitus. JAMA Intern Med 2013;173:1300–6.
52. de Galan BE, Zoungas S, Chalmers I, et al. Cognitive function and risks of cardiovascular disease and hypoglycaemia in patients with type 2 diabetes: the action in diabetes and vascular disease: preterax and Diamicron modified release controlled Evaluation (ADVANCE) trial. Diabetologia 2009;52:2328–36.
53. Punthakee Z, Miller ME, Launer LJ, et al. Poor cognitive function and risk of severe hypoglycemia in type 2 diabetes—post hoc epidemiologic analysis of the ACCORD trial. Diabetes Care 2012;35:787–93.
54. Searle SD, Rockwood K. Frailty and the risk of cognitive impairment. Alzheimers Res Ther 2015;7:54.
55. Lafortune L, Martin S, Kelly S, et al. Behavioural risk factors in mid-life associated with successful ageing, disability, dementia and frailty in later life: a rapid systematic review. PLoS One 2016;11:e0144405.
56. Fukazawa R, Hanyu H, Sato T, et al. Subgroups of Alzheimer's disease associated with diabetes mellitus based on brain imaging. Dement Geriatr Cogn Disord 2013;35:280–90.
57. Hirose D, Hanyu H, Fukasawa R, et al. Frailty in diabetes-related dementia. Geriatr Gerontol Int 2016;16:653–5.
58. Kelaiditi E, Cesari M, Canevelli M, et al. Cognitive frailty: rational and definition from an (IANA/IAGG) international consensus group. J Nutr Health Aging 2013; 17:726–34.
59. Bunn F, Burn AM, Robinson L, et al. Healthcare organisation and delivery for people with dementia and comorbidity: a qualitative study exploring the views of patients, carers and professionals. BMJ Open 2017;7:e013067.

Managing Diabetes and Dementia

Sathya Reddy, MD[a],*, Ardeshir Hashmi, MD, FACP[b]

KEYWORDS

- Dementia ● Diabetes ● Older adults ● Diabetes management

KEY POINTS

- Dementia and diabetes are both growing in prevalence in the older population.
- There is an increased risk of dementia in older adults with diabetes.
- Treatment should be individualized for older adults, keeping in mind factors such as age, comorbidities, and the patient's level of functioning in activities of daily living, instrumental activities of daily living, and cognitive domains.

INTRODUCTION

The incidence of type 2 diabetes increases with age. In 2017, the US Centers for Disease Control and Prevention estimated that 30 million individuals, or 9.4% of the US population, had diabetes. About 23.1 million people more than 65 years of age have prediabetes[1] (**Table 1**). Dementia is another condition that increases in incidence with age. The prevalence of dementia worldwide was 46.7 million in 2015 and is expected to double in the next couple of decades.[2] Diabetes and dementia are both common in older adults and increase with age, so it is not surprising that the data from the Department of Veterans' Affairs shows that the prevalence of dementia and cognitive impairment in adults with diabetes was 13.1% for adults aged 65 to 74 years, and 24.2% for adults 75 years of age and older.[3] Diabetes is an important risk factor for dementia, especially for Alzheimer and vascular dementias; there is a 1.5-fold to 2-fold increase in dementia for people with type 2 diabetes.[4,5]

Having cognitive dysfunction can affect the care of patients with diabetes in a variety of ways. Active patient involvement is needed in the care of diabetes, whether it is modifying diet, carbohydrate counting, taking medications, or exercising.[6] Depending on the level of dementia, cognitive impairment can affect the person's ability to perform some or all of these tasks. Thus, it is increasingly important to address cognitive dysfunction in patients with diabetes.

[a] Cleveland Clinic, 5700 Cooper Foster Park Road, Lorain, OH 44053, USA; [b] Cleveland Clinic, Center for Geriatric Medicine, 9500 Euclid Avenue, X10, Cleveland, OH 44195, USA
* Corresponding author.
E-mail address: Reddys3@ccf.org

Clin Geriatr Med 36 (2020) 419–429
https://doi.org/10.1016/j.cger.2020.04.003
0749-0690/20/© 2020 Elsevier Inc. All rights reserved.

geriatric.theclinics.com

Table 1
Diabetes and prediabetes

Diabetes Fast Facts	Prediabetes Fast Facts
• Total: 30.3 million people have diabetes (9.4% of the US population) • Diagnosed: 23.1 million people • Undiagnosed: 7.2 million people	• Total: 84.1 million adults aged 18 y or older have prediabetes (33.9% of the adult US population) • 65 y or older: 23.1 million adults aged 65 y or older have prediabetes

From Centers for Disease Control and Prevention. National diabetes statistics report, 2017. Atlanta, GA: Centers for Disease Control and Prevention, US Department of Health and Human Services; 2017.

RISK FACTORS FOR COGNITIVE DYSFUNCTION IN DIABETES

Diabetes is an important risk factor for Alzheimer and vascular dementia. Several studies have shown increased risk of dementia in older adults with type 2 diabetes.[7] Specific risk factors to assess include hyperglycemia, hypoglycemia, and depression.

Hyperglycemia

Studies have shown that having long-standing and poorly controlled diabetes predisposes to an increased risk for cognitive decline. This cognitive decline is also faster than in patients without diabetes.[8–10] Hyperglycemia can lead to osmotic insults and oxidative stress, and an increase in levels of advance glycosylated end products leads to brain microvascular changes and neuronal toxicity.[11]

Hypoglycemia

Some studies have shown that hypoglycemic episodes increase the risk of dementia. Severe hypoglycemia can be associated with a faster cognitive decline and with poorer initial cognitive ability.[3,12] Older adults with cognitive impairment can have a 2-fold increase in hypoglycemia; likewise, hypoglycemia can accelerate cognitive decline.[13] Hypoglycemia is also linked to delirium and fall risk. Hypoglycemic unawareness is also progressively common in older age[14] (discussed by Byron J. Hoogwerf's article, "Hypoglycemia in the Older Patient"; and Alan Sinclair and Ahmed Abdelhafiz's article, "Cognitive Dysfunction in Older Adults with Type 2 Diabetes: Links, Risks, and Clinical Implications," in this issue).

Intense control of diabetes has not been shown to decrease the risk of dementia. Action to Control Cardiovascular Risk in Diabetes (ACCORD)- Memory in Diabetes (MIND) and ACCORDION MIND, a substudy of the ACCORD trial (which showed increased mortality with intensive glucose control[15]), showed that intensive glucose level–lowering treatment over 40 months and 80 months respectively, in persons older than 55 years with type 2 diabetes, did not show any cognitive benefit.[16] Despite this, one-quarter of all US older adults with diabetes are on intensive control regimens with high hypoglycemic risk counter to guideline recommendations.[17]

Depression

Diabetes and depression are very common in the general population. Up to 25% of patients with type 2 diabetes have comorbid depression. The prevalence of depression is 31% in patients older than 65 years versus 21% in those younger than 65 years.[18] Identifying and treating depression in patients with diabetes is important because it can affect self-care of diabetes. Studies have shown that patients with type 2 diabetes and depression may have higher risk of developing dementia.[19] A 10-year dementia risk score identifies depression as one of the risk factors for dementia.[20]

HOW TO IDENTIFY COGNITIVE DYSFUNCTION

It is difficult to identify subtle changes in memory. Patients with early memory loss and a simple medication regimen may function well and cognitive impairment may be difficult to identify. Current guidelines recommend testing for patients more than 65 years of age with diabetes for memory loss. Mini-Cog[21] is a short, time-efficient screening test useful in a busy practice to identify cognitive impairment. Various other tests, such as the Montreal cognitive assessment (MoCA)[22] and the Mini Mental State Examination (MMSE),[23] are also useful screening tools to identify memory loss.

Although screening is challenging because of time constraints, screening should be performed, especially if there are symptoms of poor control of diabetes in patients who were previously well controlled or who are unable to recall medications or missing appointments.[11] Considering a referral to a geriatrician or neurologist may be appropriate for more in-depth evaluation and characterization of underlying cognitive impairment.

IMPACT OF COGNITIVE DYSFUNCTION ON DIABETES MANAGEMENT

Patients with cognitive impairment are at increased risk of developing both hypoglycemia and hyperglycemia. Hypoglycemia can have bidirectional impact: it increases the risk of dementia, and dementia then increases the risk of hypoglycemia.[11]

Patients with cognitive dysfunction have poorly controlled diabetes because they are unable to perform self-care tasks. For example, they may forget to take medication or administer insulin, or may take a wrong dose and forget to eat meals. This possibility increases the risk of developing serious episodes of hypoglycemia and hyperglycemia. For this reason, recent guidelines include screening adults 65 years of age and older for dementia and also tailoring treatment to prevent these swings in blood glucose levels.[11]

INDIVIDUALIZED GLYCEMIC GOAL SETTING

Most of the guidelines in management of diabetes take into account the cognitive ability, life expectancy, and the overall health of patients along with their comorbidities. Older adults who are otherwise healthy with few coexisting chronic illnesses and intact cognitive function and functional status should have lower glycemic goals (hemoglobin A1c [HbA1c] <7.5%).[6]

Individuals with chronic coexisting illness and cognitive impairment and/or functional dependence should have less stringent goals (HbA1c <8%–8.5%). Also, glycemic goals for some older adults might reasonably be relaxed as part of individualized care, but symptoms related to hypoglycemia or risk of acute hyperglycemia complications should be avoided.[6] Of note, given wide glycemic level excursions and comorbidities that decrease red blood cell circulation (on which the HbA1c depends), such as iron deficiency anemia, erythropoietin use, metabolic acidosis, polycythemia, and other hemoglobinopathies, HbA1c should not be the sole means of assessing glycemic control in the elderly.[14] The advent of technological advances with continuous home glucose monitoring may help address this in the near future.[24] Examples of medications for diabetes are listed in **Table 2**.

Table 2
Medications for treatment of diabetes

Medication Class	Cost	Risk of Hypoglycemia	Renal Dosage Adjustment	Side Effects
Biguanides	Low	Low	Contraindicated in GFR <30 mL/min	GI side effects nausea, vomiting, diarrhea
Thiazolidinediones	Low	Low	Not recommended in renal impairment	Can cause edema, avoid in CHF Bladder cancer concerns for pioglitazone
Meglitinides	High	High	Avoid in renal impairment	Patients with high postprandial sugar levels may benefit from it. Can skip dose if missing meal. Multidosing regimen may add to pill burden
Sulfonylureas	Low	High	Use caution in renal impairment	Avoid long-acting medications such as glyburide in elderly (Beers criteria)
GLP-1 receptor agonist	High	Low	Not recommended in GFR <30 mL/min	Nausea and vomiting, weight loss Avoid in elderly patients who are thin and frail
DPP-4 inhibitors	High	Low	Can be used in CKD	Well tolerated and once-a-day regimen. Weight neutral
SGLT2 inhibitors	High	Low	Helpful in diabetic nephropathy and in secondary prevention of CVD	Risk of limb amputation with canagliflozin Increased risk of UTI, yeast infections, Fournier gangrene
Insulin	High	High	Needs to be titrated to efficacy. Dosage can be decreased in renal insufficiency	Simpler dosing leads to reduced hypoglycemia and hyperglycemia

Abbreviations: CHF, congestive heart failure; CKD, chronic kidney disease; CVD, cardiovascular disease; DPP-4, dipeptidyl peptidase-4; GFR, glomerular filtration rate; GI, gastrointestinal; GLP-1, glucagonlike peptide 1; SGLT2, sodium-glucose transport protein 2; UTI, urinary tract infection.

MANAGEMENT OF DIABETES: CLINICAL CASE SIMULATIONS

Diabetes management should include treatment with lifestyle modification, diet, and exercise. However, special consideration should be given to treatment of older adults with different levels of functional and cognitive impairment. The following 3 cases show treatment options relevant to each patient's respective localization on the activities of daily living (ADL) and cognition spectrum. An overall framework for approaching any of these clinical case scenarios can be the 4M (what matters most, mentation, mobility and medications) model currently being embraced by the age-friendly health system movement across the United States.[25]

What matters most to patients are their overall goals of care; that is, what defines their quality of life. These specific patient goals are the "North Star" to guide the approach to personalized diabetes management. All advice and interventions should be aimed toward helping patients achieve their life goals. These goals are in turn significantly influenced by the Ms of mentation and mobility. Dementia is an entire spectrum, as clinically described by the functional assessment staging test,[26] which depicts progressive IADL (instrumental ADL) and ADL dependence with each successive stage of dementia. Under mobility lies frailty, which is pictorially depicted by the Clinical Frailty Scale,[27] which can also serve as a useful educational tool for patients and families to visually observe where they are on the frailty continuum. These progressive stages of dementia and frailty and associated loss of independence have a direct bearing on patients' ability to autonomously manage their diabetes. This scale also determines the level of in-home support they will need to achieve optimal diabetes outcomes.

Case 1

An 80-year-old male patient comes to the office for a Medicare wellness examination. He has a history of well-controlled diabetes mellitus type 2 for more than 10 years, hypertension (HTN), and hypercholesterolemia. He has no history of coronary artery disease (CAD) or cerebrovascular accident. The patient lives alone and is independent with all of his ADL.

Medications

- Glyburide 5 mg daily
- Atorvastatin 40 mg daily
- Lisinopril 20 mg daily

Physical examination

- Vitals: blood pressure: 130/60 mm Hg, with no orthostatic changes. Pulse, 85 beats/min; respiratory rate, 18 breaths/min; weight, 68 kg (150 lb); and height, 170 cm (5 feet 7 inches)
- Chest/cardiovascular/abdomen examination unremarkable
- Neurologic: no focal deficits, monofilament test negative
- Mental status: MoCA is 27/30

Laboratory tests

- Lipid profile: total cholesterol, 140 mg/dL; high-density lipoprotein, 50 mg/dL; low-density lipoprotein, 80 mg/dL
- HbA1c: 6.0%
- Complete blood count (CBC): normal
- Thyroid-stimulating hormone (TSH): 3.5 mU/L

- Basic metabolic panel (BMP) electrolytes are normal; blood urea nitrogen (BUN)/ creatinine (Cr), 20/1.1
- Urine albumin/Cr ratio less than 12 μg/mg

What are your recommendations for this patient? In case 1, the patient is community dwelling, functionally independent, with no evidence of cognitive impairment. This situation represents autonomy in engaging with diabetes management with minimal external supports required in the home setting. The fourth M, medication, is appropriately adjusted as a preemptive measure in discontinuing the glyburide to counter the hypoglycemic risk potential. The extremely good HbA1c should cause suspicious of episodic asymptomatic hypoglycemia. The clinician should check for midday hypoglycemia and make appropriate medication adjustments. As cases 2 and 3 show, with progressive cognitive and functional decline, the approach to clinical management needs to adapt accordingly.

Case 2

A 75-year-old woman with past medical history of 30 years of well-controlled type 2 diabetes, HTN, hypercholesterolemia, CAD, chronic kidney disease, diabetic neuropathy, osteoarthritis, and macular degeneration comes to the office for routine follow-up. You notice in the chart that the patient has been missing appointments, despite previously being regular with office visits. The patient did not bring her glucose log and is unable to recall her home blood sugar readings. The patient says that she had some low readings but cannot remember their values.

She lives with her husband, who is here for the appointment as well. She has a daughter who lives nearby. Her husband says he noticed that she has been more forgetful recently, but he says she is managing her medications and does not like him interfering with her routine. He notices she has been repeating things more often and has not been cooking as much, resulting in the couple eating out more often. In addition, he reports she is having difficulty with her vision. On review of the electronic medical record, she has had 2 emergency room visits for episodes of hypoglycemia in the past month.

Medications

Metformin, 500 mg twice daily
Insulin glargine, 20 units at bedtime
Regular insulin, 5 units with meals
Losartan, 50 mg daily
Pravastatin, 20 mg
Atenolol, 25 mg daily
Eye vitamins, 1 capsule daily
Acetaminophen (for arthritis), 1 tablet daily

After calling the pharmacy, you notice she has not filled her atenolol or metformin. She also has not been taking her insulin correctly, and sometimes is having trouble with self-administration of insulin.

Physical examination

General: she looks poorly kempt and disheveled
Vitals: blood pressure, 160/80 mm Hg; heart rate (HR), 84 beats/min; respiration rate, 20 breaths/min; weight, 68 kg (150 lb; a 4.5-kg [10 lb] decrease in the past 6 months)

Remainder of the examination was unremarkable except for:

Extremities: posterior tibial and dorsalis pedis pulses 2+, decreased sensation with monofilament testing. Hands show osteoarthritic changes

Mental status: MoCA 18/30

Laboratory tests

HbA1c: 9.2%

Blood glucose: 284 mg/dL

Bun/Cr: 25/1.3

Liver enzymes are normal

CBC, TSH, and vitamin B_{12} levels are normal

What are your recommendations for this patient? This patient has microvascular and macrovascular complications related to diabetes. Having hyperglycemic and hypoglycemic episodes is associated bidirectionally with dementia risk. The high HbA1c level does not necessarily rule out hypoglycemic episodes. The patient has cognitive impairment based on history and memory testing. Dementia increases hypoglycemia risk. Cognitive impairment affects adherence to appropriate diet and medications. She has other comorbidities, including vision impairment, gait abnormality, and polypharmacy.

A multidisciplinary approach involving the social worker, arranging home meal delivery through a local community program, and arranging home delivery of medications through a prepackaged pill pack will ensure a safer environment for the patient. Including the family in assisting with reminders for meals, medications, and tracking her daily blood sugar levels is important. A practically feasible goal should be set of her walking for 5 to 10 minutes a couple of times a day to improve her activity level. Her medications were reviewed and recommendations to simplify her medication regimen were made. Her short-acting insulin was stopped to decrease the risk of hypoglycemia. Simplification of insulin regimens from multiple-dose insulin regimens to once-daily insulin has been shown to decrease hypoglycemic episodes as well as diabetes-related distress scores.[28]

Her long-acting insulin was changed from vial to pens for ease of insulin administration. Timing of long-acting insulin administration was changed to the morning, again as a countermeasure to prevent fasting hypoglycemia and also because postprandial glucose levels contribute more to overall geriatric hyperglycemia than fasting glucose.[29]

If more than 50% of glucose values are greater than the goal, the dose of basal insulin should be increased by 2 to 3 units every 7 to 10 days, titrated to a fasting glucose range of 90 to 150 mg/dL in older adults. If 2 or more fasting values are less than 80 mg/dL, basal insulin should be decreased by 2 units. Noninsulin agents should be adjusted based on postprandial glucose levels. Her target HbA1c was set to less than 8.5%.

Progressive cognitive decline has affected this patient's ability to independently monitor glycemic levels, take measures to counter hypoglycemia, manage a complex medication regimen, and adhere to a nutrition plan or sustain an exercise program. The resultant increased level of IADL dependence may necessitate a discussion with patient and family about a potential transition to a higher level of care; for example, an assisted living facility.

The advantages and disadvantages of this transition would need to be carefully considered; Although help with medication regimen administration and glucose monitoring may be optimized, the patient's control over diet may be compromised in an institutional setting.[14] In addition, communication between the assisted living and the patient's primary care physician and/or endocrinologist team will be critical. In this instance, fortuitously available family support was optimized.

Two-week follow-up visit Two weeks later, the patient had gained 0.9 kg (2 lb) and has had no new episodes of hypoglycemia. Her daughter is also present at this appointment. They bring in her glucose log, which shows that they have been regularly checking her levels once a day, with morning readings around 140 to 150 mg/dL. There are occasional checks before dinner, with levels around 170 to 200 mg/dL. The patient seems more coherent and less anxious. Her computed tomography brain imaging shows microvascular changes only. She was also started on donepezil for her dementia.

Three-month follow-up visit Three months later she was tolerating donepezil 5 mg well, and her memory seems stable per family accounts. Her HbA1c is now 7.8%. Her weight is stable at 71 kg (156 lb).

Case 3

An 88-year-old woman with a past medical history of DM, HTN, hypercholesterolemia, and severe dementia needs help with all of her ADL. She has recently moved into a long-term care facility, and you are the physician taking care of her there.

On your first visit you notice that she is pleasant and alert, but mumbling words and not very communicative. She is mostly bed bound but comes out to the dining room for meals. She does not appear in distress but cannot verbalize any concerns. The nurses note that she seems pleasant and has no behavioral concerns.

Medications

Metformin, 500 mg twice daily
Simvastatin, 10 mg daily
Donepezil, 5 mg
Enalapril, 5 mg daily

Physical examination

Vitals: blood pressure 134/58 mm Hg; HR, 64 beats/min; weight 56 kg (124 lb)
Remainder of the examination was unremarkable except for:
Neurology: the patient is not oriented to place, person, or time, and she mumbles words that are not recognizable

Laboratory tests

BMP and CBC are unremarkable: BUN, 25 mg/dL; Cr, 1.6 mg/dL; estimated glomerular filtration rate (eGFR), 28 mL/min
Vitamin B_{12} and TSH levels are normal
HbA1c: 7.4%

What are your recommendations for this patient? This patient has severe dementia affecting all her ADL. Goals of care should be discussed with her family. Prevention of vascular complications of diabetes is not a long-term goal. Palliative care and symptom alleviation may be appropriate for this patient. Metformin may also have to be held because of the patient's reduced eGFR. Simvastatin, Donepezil, and Metformin could be discontinued to decrease overall pill burden and her glycemic and metabolic control simultaneously monitored. The goal is to avoid symptomatic hyperglycemia and maintain hydration and electrolyte status.

Unless the care management plan is aligned with the patient's advanced clinical debility and overall goals of care, the vicious cycle of avoidable hospital transfers discordant with patient's wishes cannot be broken. Given advanced stages of cognitive and functional decline, overall life expectancy must be considered, and the focus should be on quality of life. Patient prioritized care with patient/family-defined health outcomes and care preferences as its core guiding philosophy is primed to revolutionize age-appropriate quality metrics for older adults with multiple comorbidities, including diabetes and dementia.[30]

SUMMARY

An aging global population has heralded the ever-growing prevalence of diabetes with concurrent dementia. Annual cognitive and functional assessments engender a clinical paradigm shift toward both early intervention and developing personalized care plans, customized to individual cognitive and functional capabilities. Integral to fostering this is a multidisciplinary team approach, including recruiting patient/family support. Simplification and deintensification of medication regimens and avoiding hypoglycemia triggers are essential. With progressive cognitive and functional impairment, discussions about potential transitions to higher care support settings, liberalization of glycemic goals, and compatibility with overall goals of care define current best practices, as well as providing a blueprint for an aging future.

DISCLOSURE

The authors have nothing to disclose.

REFERENCES

1. Centers for Disease control and Prevention. National diabetes statistics report, 2017. Atlanta (GA): Centers for Disease Control and Prevention, US Department of Health and Human Services; 2017.
2. Prince M, Wilmo A, Guerchet M, et al. World Alzheimer report 2015: the global impact of dementia. Alzheimers Dis Int 2015.
3. Feil DG, Rajan M, Soroka O, et al. Risk of hypoglycemia in older veterans with dementia and cognitive impairment: implications for practice and policy. J Am Geriatr Soc 2011;59(12):2263–72.
4. Ott A, Stolk RP, van Harskamp F, et al. Diabetes mellitus and the risk of dementia: the Rotterdam Study. Neurology 1999;53(9):1937–42.
5. Peila R, Rodriguez BL, Launer LJ, Honolulu-Asia Aging Study. Type 2 diabetes, APOE gene, and the RIsk for dementia and related pathologies. Diabetes 2002;51(4):1256–62.
6. American Diabetes Association. 12. Older adults: standards of medical care in diabetes-2019. Diabetes Care 2019;42(Suppl 1):S139–47.
7. Mayeda ER, Whitmer RA, Yaffe K. Diabetes and cognition. Clin Geriatr Med 2015; 31(1):101–15, ix.
8. Yaffe K1 FC, Hamilton N, Schwartz AV, et al. Diabetes, glucose control, and 9-year cognitive decline among older adults without dementia. Arch Neurol 2012; 69(9):1770–5.
9. Tuligenga RH, Dugravot A, Tabák A, et al. Midlife type 2 diabetes and poor glycaemic control as risk factors for cognitive decline in early old age: a post-hoc

analysis of the Whitehall II cohort study. Lancet Diabetes Endocrinol 2014;2(3): 228–35.

10. Spauwen PJ1 KS, Verhey FR, Stehouwer CD, et al. Effects of type 2 diabetes on 12-year cognitive change: results from the Maastricht Aging Study. Diabetes Care 2013;36(6):1554–61.

11. Munshi MN. Cognitive dysfunction in older adults with diabetes: what a clinician needs to know. Diabetes Care 2017;40(4):461–7.

12. Lin CH, Sheu WH. Hypoglycaemic episodes and risk of dementia in diabetes mellitus: 7-year follow-up study. J Intern Med 2013;273(1):102–10.

13. Feinkohl I, Aung PP, Keller M, et al, Edinburgh Type 2 Diabetes Study (ET2DS) Investigators. Severe hypoglycemia and cognitive decline in older people with type 2 diabetes: the Edinburgh type 2 diabetes study. Diabetes Care 2014; 37(2):507–15.

14. Leung E, Wongrakpanich S, Munshi MN. Diabetes management in the elderly. Diabetes Spectr 2018;31(3):245–53. https://doi.org/10.2337/ds18-0033.

15. Action to Control Cardiovascular Risk in Diabetes Study Group, Gerstein HC, Miller ME, Byington RP, et al. Effects of intensive glucose lowering in type 2 diabetes. N Engl J Med 2008;358(24):2545–59.

16. Murray AM, Hsu FC, Williamson JD, et al, Action to Control Cardiovascular Risk in Diabetes Follow-On Memory in Diabetes (ACCORDION MIND) Investigators. ACCORDION MIND: results of the observational extension of the ACCORD MIND randomised trial. Diabetologia 2017;60(1):69–80.

17. Arnold SV, Lipska KJ, Wang J, et al. Use of intensive glycemic management in older adults with diabetes mellitus. J Am Geriatr Soc 2018;66(6):1190–4.

18. Katona W, Pedersen HS, Ribe AR, et al. Effect of depression and diabetes mellitus on the risk for dementia: a national population-based cohort study. JAMA Psychiatry 2015;72(6):612–9.

19. Katon W, Lyles CR, Parker MM, et al. Association of depression with increased risk of dementia in patients with type 2 diabetes: the Diabetes and Aging Study. Arch Gen Psychiatry 2012;69(4):410–7.

20. Exalto LG, Biessels GJ, Karter AJ, et al. Risk score for prediction of 10 year dementia risk in individuals with type 2 diabetes: a cohort study. Lancet Diabetes Endocrinol 2013;1(3):183–90.

21. Sinclair AJ, Gadsby R, Hilson R, et al. Brief report: use of the Mini-Cog as a screening tool for cognitive impairment in diabetes in primary care. Diabetes Res Clin Pract 2013;100(1):23–5.

22. Nasreddine ZS, Phillips NA, Bedirian V, et al. The Montreal Cognitive Assessment, MoCA: a brief screening tool for mild cognitive impairment. J Am Geriatr Soc 2005;53(4):695–9.

23. Folstein MF, Folstein SE, McHugh P. Mini Mental State: a practical method for grading the cognitive state of patients for the clinician. J Psychiatr Res 1975; 12(3):189–98.

24. Ruedy KJ, Parkin CG, Riddlesworth TD, Graham C for the DIAMOND Study Group. Continuous glucose monitoring in older patients with Type I and Type II Diabetes using multiple daily injections of Insulin: results from the Diamind trial. J Diabetes Sci Technol 2017;11(6):1138–46.

25. Allen K, Ouslander JG. Age-friendly health systems: their time has come. J Am Geriatr Soc 2017;66(1):19–21.

26. Sclan SG, Reisberg B. Functional assessment staging (FAST) in Alzheimer's disease: reliability, validity, and ordinality. Int Psychogeriatr 1992;4(Suppl 1):55–69.

27. Rockwood K, Song X, MacKnight C, et al. A global clinical measure of fitness and frailty in elderly people. CMAJ 2005;173(5):489–95.
28. Munshi MN, Slyne C, Segal AR, et al. Simplification of insulin regimen in older adults and risk of hypoglycemia. JAMA Intern Med 2016;176(7):1023–5.
29. Munshi MN, Pandya N, Umpierrez GE, et al. Contributions of basal and prandial hyperglycemia to total hyperglycemia in older and younger adults with type 2 diabetes mellitus. J Am Geriatr Soc 2013;61(4):535–41.
30. Tinetti ME, Esterson J, Ferris R, et al. Patient priority-directed decision making and care for older adults with multiple chronic conditions. Clin Geriatr Med 2016;32(2):261–75.

Renal Evaluation and Protection

Rawan Amir, MBBS[a], Sara Suhl, BS[b], Charles M. Alexander, MD[c],*

KEYWORDS

- Diabetic nephropathy • Type 2 diabetes • Albuminuria • Chronic kidney disease

KEY POINTS

- To emphasize the appropriate screening and evaluation of diabetic nephropathy in the elderly population.
- To highlight the differences in recommendations of treatment of comorbidities in elderly patients with diabetes versus those of their younger counterparts.
- To raise awareness of the renoprotective benefits of certain oral antihyperglycemic agents, particularly sodium-glucose cotransporter-2 inhibitors (SGLT-2i) and glucagon-like peptide-1 receptor agonists (GLP-1RA).

In the 1960s, the diagnosis of diabetic nephropathy was equivalent to being diagnosed with a terminal disease. Little was understood about the disease process at the time; however, physicians were aware that proteinuria associated with elevated blood sugar levels was associated with rapid progression of renal dysfunction. They also noted that patients diagnosed with diabetes at a younger age were more likely to develop diabetic nephropathy than those diagnosed at later stages in life. The grim outcome of diabetic nephropathy was that once a patient was found to have persistent proteinuria, they almost certainly progressed to end-stage renal disease (ESRD); nearly 50% found to have proteinuria developed ESRD within a decade.[1] However, over time, physicians gained a better understanding of the disease itself and have since been able to better evaluate, monitor, and treat diabetic nephropathy, a common sequela of the disease of the twenty-first century, diabetes.

One cannot bundle all diabetic nephropathy patients into one group. There are those with minimal symptoms and well-preserved renal function and those with overt signs and symptoms of renal failure requiring renal-replacement therapy. To distinguish patients of varying severity levels of the disease and to ensure a unanimous

a Central Michigan University, College of Medicine, Dept of Medicine, 1000 Houghton Ave, Saginaw, MI 48602, USA; b dQ&A Diabetes Research, 804 Haight Street, San Francisco, CA 94117, USA; c Alexander Associates LLC, PO Box 351, Gwynedd Valley, PA 19437, USA
* Corresponding author.
E-mail address: cmalexandermd@gmail.com

Clin Geriatr Med 36 (2020) 431–445
https://doi.org/10.1016/j.cger.2020.04.004
0749-0690/20/© 2020 Elsevier Inc. All rights reserved.

opinion regarding the degree of diabetic nephropathy among all physicians, a diabetic nephropathy classification system was created.

The classification recommended by the Joint Committee on Diabetic Nephropathy in 2014 divides this disease into five distinct categories based on albumin excretion (albumin to creatinine ratio [ACR]) and estimated glomerular filtration rate (eGFR). The initial stage is prenephropathy with normal albuminuria (ACR <30 mg/g) and an eGFR of 30 mL/min/1.73 m^2 or more; it is followed by the second category of incipient nephropathy characterized by microalbuminuria (ACR 30–299 mg/g) and eGFR of 30 mL/min/1.73 m^2 or more. This stage is followed by the third category of overt nephropathy, where the patient has macroalbuminuria (ACR of 300 mg/g or more) or with persistent proteinuria of 0.5 g or more associated with a minimal eGFR of 30 mL/min/1.73 m^2. The fourth category is kidney failure, which includes any patient with diabetic nephropathy and an eGFR less than 30 mL/min/1.73 m^2. The fifth and final category is renal-replacement therapy, which involves any patient with diabetic nephropathy requiring either dialysis or renal transplant.[2,3]

Another more frequently used classification of chronic kidney disease (CKD), in general, categorizes patients according to their eGFR and degree of albuminuria. Patients are classified according to their eGFR from G1-G5 and according to their ACR from A1-A3 (**Fig. 1**).

To estimate the GFR and hence classify patients without the need for 24-hour urine collection, multiple formulas have been created. In the past, the most commonly used formula worldwide was the Cockcroft-Gault formula developed in 1973 using data

KDIGO 2012				Persistent albuminuria categories Description and range		
				A1	A2	A3
				Normal to mildly increased	Moderately increased	Severely increased
				<30 mg/g <3 mg/mmol	30-300 mg/g 3-30 mg/mmol	>300 mg/g >30 mg/mmol
GFR categories (ml/min/ 1.73 m^2) Description and range	G1	Normal or high	≥90			
	G2	Mildly decreased	60-89			
	G3a	Mildly to moderately decreased	45-59			
	G3b	Moderately to severely decreased	30-44			
	G4	Severely decreased	15-29			
	G5	Kidney failure	<15			

Green: low risk (if no other markers of kidney disease, no CKD); Yellow: moderately increased risk; Orange: high risk; Red, very high risk.

Fig. 1. Prognosis of CKD by GFR and albuminuria category. (*From* Kidney Disease: Improving Global Outcomes (KDIGO). 2012 clinical practice guideline for the evaluation and management of chronic kidney disease. Available at: https://kdigo.org/wp-content/uploads/2017/02/KDIGO_2012_CKD_GL.pdf; with permission.)

from 249 men. It is not adjusted for body surface area and no longer recommended for use because it has not been expressed using standardized creatinine values. Another estimating equation for GFR is the Modification of Diet and Renal Disease (MDRD) formula. More recently, the Chronic Kidney Disease Epidemiology Collaboration equation was created and has proven to be somewhat more precise than MDRD, especially with regard to estimating GFR in those with a GFR more than 60 mm/min/1.73 m^2 and is equally accurate as MDRD in estimating GFR in those with a GFR less than 60 mL/min/1.73 m^2.[4] What these formulas have failed to represent accurately is the eGFR in the elderly population. These equations may overestimate the GFR in this subset of patients. Therefore, when estimating GFR in elderly patients, it is vital to use equations that consider age as an independent variable. Both the MDRD and Chronic Kidney Disease Epidemiology Collaboration equations were subsequently modified to include patients' age.

Serum creatinine is used to estimate GFR. However, two large meta-analyses concluded that creatinine is inferior to cystatin C when it comes to assessing renal function. Although cystatin C is more accurate, it is much more expensive and not as readily available as creatinine in many medical centers. Therefore, the only clear recommendation to use cystatin C nowadays is for the confirmation of CKD in patients who lack any other indicative markers of kidney dysfunction.[5]

Similar to any other organ in the body, the kidneys are affected by the aging process. These changes start to occur in the third decade of life and continue to progress gradually. These changes affect all individuals regardless of the presence or absence of concomitant comorbidities; any present comorbidities, however, can affect the rate and severity of decline in renal function. Functional renal age-related changes are represented by a steady reduction in GFR[6]; yet, the rate of decline is still a topic of debate. The MDRD study reports declines at a rate of 3.8 mL/min/year/1.73 m^2, yet other studies report rates of 0.4 mL/min/year/1.73 m^2 in the Netherlands.[7] Now, the question that is always raised is whether or not the method used in measuring the GFR accurately represents that of the aging population. Despite the gold standard for measuring GFR being 24-hour clearance of inulin or creatinine, one of the estimating equations for GFR based on serum creatinine levels and age is frequently used. However, creatinine production, and hence serum levels, rely on muscle mass, which is significantly reduced in the elderly population as part of the normal aging process. Another point of concern that led to questioning eGFR is the hyperbolic relationship between creatinine and GFR, leading to reduced sensitivity, particularly when the GFR is still greater than 50 mL/min/1.73 m^2.[8] These questions eventually led to the development of specific formulas to more accurately estimate the GFR in those older than 70 years.

Macroscopic changes seen in the aging kidney include a reduction in the overall volume of the kidney and an increase in renal cysts. Kidney size has been shown to have an inverse relationship with age. On average, a reduction of around 16 cm^3 per decade is expected.[9] Other studies report an even larger reduction in kidney size at around 22 cm^3 per decade. This study not only examined the rate of reduction in renal size but further studied the anatomy of the kidneys throughout the aging process only to discover that as we age, the renal cortex loses mass but is compensated by growth of the renal medulla. This discovery explains the lack of change in overall renal size because medullary growth is compensating for cortical loss. But with time, decompensation occurs, and reduction in renal size begins to be noted; this typically occurs around the age of 50 years.[10] Another noticeable macroscopic renal age-related change is the increase in the number and size of simple renal cysts, more often involving cortical cysts as opposed to medullary, and more frequently in males than females.[11]

As the life expectancy of the general population increases, health problems of the elderly population are more commonly encountered. Diabetic nephropathy per se is becoming a condition primarily in the elderly population. The National Health and Nutrition Examination Survey done in 2005 to 2008 concluded that diabetes mellitus affects 3.7% of adults between the age of 20 and 44 years, 13.7% of adults between 45 and 64 years of age, and up to 26.9% of adults older than 65 years of age. Many institutes including the Centers for Disease Control and Prevention estimate that the prevalence of diabetes is going to double over the next 20 years not because of an increase in incidence, but because of the increase in life expectancy. Therefore, diabetes mellitus and diabetic nephropathy are going to be encountered more frequently in patients older than the age of 65.[12]

As diabetic nephropathy starts affecting this population that tends to have multiple comorbidities, the actual pathogenesis of the disease itself is starting to change. The classic presentation of Kimmelstiel-Wilson nodules on renal biopsy is less commonly present, and current pathology is often more suggestive of hypertension and ischemic changes, possibly because of atherosclerosis. As the causative factors of the disease change, the management of diabetic nephropathy in the elderly population also must change.

To fully appreciate and comprehend the differences in management between diabetic nephropathy in the general population and diabetic nephropathy in the elderly population, we must first review the guidelines for management of diabetic nephropathy in the general population. The current guidelines for screening and treatment of diabetic nephropathy in the general population are from the National Kidney Foundation and the American Diabetes Association. It is recommended that the urine ACR be performed on an annual basis to screen patients at risk of developing diabetic nephropathy.[13–15]

It is recommended that an angiotensin-converting enzyme inhibitor or an angiotensin receptor blocker, also known as renin-angiotensin-aldosterone system (RAAS) blockers, be the primary pharmacologic agent for those with diabetic nephropathy because it may help in the control of albuminuria while also controlling blood pressure. These agents are recommended to be used in patients with an ACR of 30 to 299 mg/g creatinine and are strongly recommended in those with a ratio equal to or greater than 300 mg/g creatinine or with a GFR less than 60 mL/min/1.73 m^2. Patients with a GFR less than 60 mL/min/1.73 m^2 must be screened for any potential complications of CKD. Those with a GFR less than 30 mL/min/1.73 m^2 must be referred to a nephrologist for consideration of potential renal-replacement therapy in the near future. These agents are recommended to be used in normotensive patients with diabetes only if the albuminuria levels are greater than 30 mg/g (recommendation of the National Kidney Foundation, level 2C).[13,14] For the goal blood pressure, in patients with diabetes with albuminuria, the target is less than 130/80, whereas it is less than 140/90 in patients without albuminuria.[14]

A low-density lipoprotein cholesterol-lowering agent, such as a statin, is suggested to be used to control hyperlipidemia in patients with diabetes.[14]

Treatment of hyperglycemia itself is preferably with a sodium-glucose cotransporter-2 inhibitor (SGLT-2i) or a glucagon-like peptide-1 receptor agonist (GLP-1RA). SGLT-2i has been shown to slow down the progression of CKD in patients with diabetes, and GLP-1RA has been shown to reduce albuminuria.[13,14]

How do these guidelines differ when it comes to the elderly population? Elderly patients are more likely to die from cardiovascular (CV) events as opposed to developing ESRD. Although better glycemic control has been proven over time to reduce the rate of development of diabetic nephropathy and other microvascular complications, there is not much evidence that shows that it reduces macrovascular or CV events, and there is the issue of competing mortality from any cause in this population. Therefore, the ideal hemoglobin A_{1C} (HbA_{1c}) target when attempting to control hyperglycemia in the elderly population remains a heated topic of debate.

Regarding control of associated comorbidities, such as hypertension, the use of RAAS blockers is the logical choice in the younger population. This is because this age group is mainly affected by type 1 diabetes, where the pathophysiology of diabetic nephropathy is microvascular in nature. Therefore, the RAAS plays an active role in hyperfiltration of proteins in the glomeruli, hence worsening the albuminuria; blockage of the system improves proteinuria and, subsequently, diabetic nephropathy. Comparing this with the pathophysiology of diabetic nephropathy in the elderly population that is more macrovascular in nature, the RAAS is playing a protective role by ensuring proper blood flow to the kidneys and preventing ischemia.[12] Multiple trials support this theory including the Aliskiren trial in type 2 diabetes using CV and renal disease end points (ALTITUDE) trial in addition to the ongoing telmisartan alone and in combination with ramipril global end point trial (On Target), which have shown that blocking the RAAS in patients with type 2 diabetes by combination therapy may be detrimental and was associated with higher rates of acute kidney injury, hypotension, and hyperkalemia.[16] Therefore, one must be wary of overtreating and too aggressively blocking the RAAS in the elderly population.

The next obvious question is, what would the target systolic blood pressure be in the elderly population. There are many trials and studies that have been done to answer this question. One large observational study of 881 patients with type 2 diabetes showed an inverse relationship between blood pressure readings and mortality in patients 75 years of age and older. They found that a reduction of 10 mm Hg and systolic and diastolic blood pressure led to a 20% and 26% increase in mortality, respectively, although in younger patients there was no significant relationship between mortality and blood pressure.[17] The Action to Control Cardiovascular Risk in Diabetes (ACCORD) trial (mean age, 62.2 years) did not show any improvement in mortality associated with blood pressure control less than 140/90, and also showed an increased incidence of renal impairment and hypokalemia with a target systolic blood pressure less than 120 mm Hg systolic compared with 140 mm Hg.[18] These findings were also strongly supported by the International Verapamil SR Trandolapril Study (INVEST; mean age, 66 years), which showed no mortality benefit when target systolic blood pressure was less than 130 mm Hg compared with those with a systolic blood pressure of 130 to 139 mm Hg.[19] Therefore, the recommended optimal systolic blood pressure for elderly patients is currently 140 mm Hg systolic.

Elderly patients are often frail and more prone to develop side effects of medications compared with the younger population. Therefore, note that when treating hypertension in elderly patients, it is preferable to start at a low dose and slowly up-titrate according to the patient's tolerance. In addition, it is important to educate the patient along with their caregivers on possible side effects of medications. Many elderly patients are placed on diuretics, whether thiazide or loop diuretics, and suffer from complications of these medications, which eventually lead to hospitalization, such as dehydration, hypotension, tachycardia, and oliguria. Patients and caregivers must be wary of the side effects and notify their physician as soon as possible to adjust the medical therapy. In addition, close monitoring of potassium and creatinine levels in patients prescribed angiotensin-converting enzyme inhibitor or angiotensin receptor blockers needs to be done.

As for control of dyslipidemia, the general consensus is that elderly patients do benefit from statin therapy, which plays a role in the reduction of CV events. The effects of statin therapy become evident quickly (within 1–2 years of initiation) with therapy; hence, it is recommended that all elderly patients start statin therapy aside from those with shortened life expectancy. Not enough data are available regarding the exact cholesterol level goals in this population currently to set clear targets. However, observational studies have shown that the highest mortality in patients older than the age of 80 years was associated with the lowest total cholesterol less than 100 mg/dL (5.5 mmol/L).[20] Multiple studies have shown that higher cholesterol levels in the later stages of life are associated with a reduction of dementia. What we can conclude in regard to treating diabetes and diabetic nephropathy is that treatment in the elderly must be individualized for each patient based on their specific characteristics and life expectancy.

Overall diet and lifestyle modification recommendations for middle-aged and elderly patients are similar. It is recommended that any patient with diabetic nephropathy limit protein consumption to 0.8 to 1.0 g/kg daily. If the eGFR is less than 60 mL/min/1.73 m^2, the daily protein intake should be reduced to even lower than 0.8 g/kg daily. The source of proteins is preferred to be plant-based as opposed to animal-based. In addition, limitation of salt intake to improve hypertension control is also recommended. It has been shown that reduction of salt intake is as effective as being on a single antihypertensive agent in controlling blood pressure levels when done appropriately. The current recommendation is to limit salt intake to 5 to 6 g/d or less if possible. Smoking is a major risk factor for CKD and diabetic nephropathy; hence, smoking cessation is recommended in patients with diabetes of all ages.[21]

So far, the discussion has revolved around diabetic nephropathy with low GFR and albuminuria. However, diabetic nephropathy in the absence of albuminuria has become increasingly recognized. With current medical advancements, rates of albuminuria have generally been decreasing in patients with diabetes. Still lacking, however, is proven medical therapy for the prevention of progression of diabetic nephropathy in the absence of albuminuria.

Diabetic nephropathy was initially believed to follow a specific path starting with normal urine albumin excretion ACR less than 30 mg/g, which progresses to moderate urine albumin excretion with ACR 30 to 300 mg/g subsequently followed by severely worsening urine albumin excretion with ACR greater than 300 mg/g. After urine albumin excretion worsened significantly, GFR would begin to fall. However, what has been noticed recently is that despite patients having lower or normal urine albumin excretion (which may be secondary to the use of RAAS antagonists), the GFR still worsened significantly regardless of ACR. This, in turn, prompted studies focusing on patients with diabetes with low GFR without elevated urine albumin excretion. One large study that reviewed data from the National Health and Nutrition Examination Survey showed that one in every six American adults with diabetes has a GFR less than 60 mL/min/1.73 m^2. What is even more surprising is that nearly half of these patients with low GFRs do not have albuminuria. They also concluded that mortality rates were trending upward in patients with diabetes with low GFR and no proteinuria, whereas improving in those with reduced GFR and ACR more than 30 mg/g.[22]

In regard to the clinical course of diabetic nephropathy in patients without albuminuria, a study following GFR and albuminuria trends in 935 patients with type 1 diabetes and 1984 with type 2 diabetes showed that patients tend to follow one of two paths. The first path represents most patients (86% with type 1 diabetes and 90% with type 2 diabetes) where an initial improvement in GFR is seen after being diagnosed with stage III CKD followed by a gradual reduction of GFR. The initial improvement in GFR may be secondary to increased treatment after diagnosis of a patient with CKD stage III. The other group encompasses patients who have a rapid decline in

GFR initially followed by either a plateau phase or a slight improvement in GFR.[23] This is to emphasize that even patients with diabetes with no albuminuria have declining GFRs more rapidly than their nondiabetic counterparts.

Most elderly patients with diabetes die from cardiac comorbidities associated with diabetes as opposed to ESRD. Patients with poorly controlled diabetes are more prone to develop cardiac complications. Reduced eGFR and high ACR are both independent risk factors for heart failure. A study published in 2018 of 5801 patients concluded that the combination of both is associated with an even higher risk. However, it is not only patients with diabetic nephropathy and high ACR who are at risk of these cardiac complications.[24] A recent study of CV disease risk in nonalbuminuric diabetic nephropathy proved that despite having a low/normal ACR, patients with diabetes with low eGFR are still more likely to suffer CV events than the general population. In a study of 18,227 patients with diabetes followed for a 5-year period with monitoring of ACR and eGFR, the authors concluded that the highest mortality was in those with low eGFR and high ACR followed by those with low eGFR and normal ACR.[25] Therefore, a large shift in focus was made to further understand CV events in patients with diabetes with variable ACRs to find the optimal treatment modality with the goal of improving patient outcomes, morbidity, and mortality.

Although metformin and sulfonylureas continue to be the most widely prescribed therapies for those with type 2 diabetes, newer drug classes have emerged with promising benefits in addition to lowering glycated HbA_{1c}. GLP-1RA and SGLT-2i have been the subject of inquiry in multiple recent CV outcome trials. Although much of these trials' focus, with one exception, was on CV end points, the microvascular and renal outcomes of these studies give insight into the renal-protective effects these drug classes may provide.[26]

GLP-1RA are a group of drugs that work by mimicking the effects of GLP-1, an incretin. GLP-1 increases insulin release while decreasing glucagon secretion, thus lowering fasting and postprandial glucose levels. GLP-1RA have proven beneficial for renal protection by reducing known risk factors, such as obesity, hypertension, hyperglycemia, and dyslipidemia. Additionally, GLP-1RA may play a direct role in renal tubular and glomerular functioning.[27] The renal outcomes of GLP-1RA were evaluated as secondary end points in four CV outcomes trials: ELIXA (Evaluation of Lixisenatide in Acute coronary syndrome), LEADER (Liraglutide Effects and Action in Diabetes: Evaluation of cardiovascular outcome Results), SUSTAIN-6 (Trial to Evaluate Cardiovascular and Other Long-term Outcomes With Semaglutide in Subjects With Type 2 Diabetes), and EXSCEL (Exenatide Study of Cardiovascular Event Lowering).

ELIXA was the first to report renal outcomes for the GLP-1RA class. The trial studied the CV and renal effects of lixisenatide, a short-acting GLP-1RA against placebo. It followed over 6000 study participants with type 2 diabetes who had experienced an acute coronary event in the last 6 months (<180 days) **(Fig. 2)**.[27]

The LEADER trial investigated CV and renal outcomes of liraglutide compared with placebo in 9340 randomized participants with type 2 diabetes and a high risk of experiencing a CV event. LEADER's prespecified renal outcome was defined as new or worsening nephropathy. This composite outcome included new onset or the persistence of macroalbuminuria, the doubling of serum creatinine with an eGFR less than or equal to 45 mL/min/1.73 m^2, the need for renal-replacement therapy, and renal death. Results from the trial showed that treatment with liraglutide reduced the renal composite outcome by 22% after 3.8 years (95% confidence interval [CI], 8%–33%; $P = .003$) of treatment, largely caused by a 26% reduction in macroalbuminuria. However, hard renal end points, such as the occurrence of end-stage kidney disease (ESKD) or renal death, were unaffected. Additionally, after

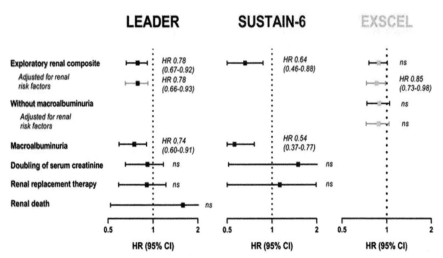

Fig. 2. Exploratory renal outcomes and their individual components in CV outcome trials. LEADER reported a composite renal outcome that consisted of new-onset persistent macro-albuminuria, persistent doubling of serum creatinine and an eGFR less than 45 mL/min/1.73 m². need for renal-replacement therapy, or renal death. Post hoc adjustments were made for change from baseline in HbA$_{1c}$, body weight, and systolic blood pressure. SUSTAIN-6 reported a composite renal outcome that consisted of new-onset persistent macroalbuminuria, persistent doubling of serum creatinine and an eGFR less than 45 mL/min/1.73 m², and need for renal-replacement therapy. No data showing adjustments for renal risk factors are available. EXSCEL reported two composite renal outcomes. The first consisted of 40% eGFR decline, need for renal-replacement therapy, or renal death. The second consisted of new-onset macroalbuminuria, 40% eGFR decline, need for renal-replacement therapy, or renal death and is depicted here. Adjustment was made for renal risk factors age, sex, ethnicity, race, region, duration of diabetes, prior history of CV event, insulin use, baseline HbA$_{1c}$, eGFR, and body mass index. CI, confidence interval; HR, hazard ratio; ns = not significant. (*From* van Baar MJB, van der Aart AB, Hoogenberg K, et al. The incretin pathway as a therapeutic target in diabetic kidney disease: a clinical focus on GLP-1 receptor agonists. Ther Adv Endocrinol Metab. 2019;10:6; with permission.)

controlling for improvements to weight, HbA$_{1C}$, and blood pressure, the LEADER trial found the renal benefits of liraglutide to be independent of glucose levels. Liraglutide also had positive effects on eGFR trajectories, with a 2% slower decline in eGFR compared with placebo. This effect was most dramatic in those with baseline renal functioning considered moderately (eGFR, 30–59 mL/min/1.73 m²) or severely (eGFR, <30 mL/min/1.73 m²) reduced. However, the number of study participants with CKD beyond stage 4 was limited. Overall, the LEADER trial proved liraglutide's safety among those in its study population and in those with CKD.[28]

The SUSTAIN-6 trial investigated CV and renal outcomes of semaglutide compared with placebo in 3297 participants with type 2 diabetes and a high risk of experiencing a CV event. Like the LEADER trial, the SUSTAIN-6 trial used a prespecified renal composite outcome that was defined as new or worsening nephropathy. This composite outcome was the same as LEADER and included new onset or the persistence of macroalbuminuria, the doubling of serum creatinine with an eGFR less than or equal to 45 mL/min/1.73 m², the need for renal-replacement therapy, and renal death. Study findings showed the renal-protective effects of semaglutide to be potentially more dramatic than liraglutide. Treatment with semaglutide resulted in a reduction of the renal composite end point by 36% after 2.1 years (95% CI, 12%–54%; P = .005) compared with placebo, with macroalbuminuria reductions of 46% and no effect on rates of ESRD or renal death. Semaglutide's composite renal outcome and macroalbuminuria reductions were 14% and 20% greater, respectively, than those of liraglutide. Unlike liraglutide, however, SUSTAIN-6 did not show that the results were independent of glucose level. Semaglutide was also deemed safe for all groups included in the study.[29]

The EXSCEL trial studied the CV and renal outcomes of exenatide. The study followed 14,752 people with type 2 diabetes, with 73% of study participants having a previous diagnosis of CV disease. Rates of ESRD and renal death were unaffected by the weekly dose of exenatide when compared with the placebo. eGFR levels and new-onset macroalbuminuria were also similar in the treatment and placebo groups. The Harmony Outcomes trial investigating albiglutide similarly found that albiglutide did not significantly affect eGFR after 16 months.[27]

Although GLP-1RA outcomes for those with CKD have not been the focus of these CV outcome trials, some insight into the drug class's effects on this group are obtained from the studies. A post hoc analysis of the ELIXA trial studying the effects of lixisenatide concluded that lixisenatide decreased urine ACR, even when controlling for changes in renal risk factors, such as weight, blood pressure, and HbA_{1C}, which may have occurred during the course of the trial. Those with baseline microalbuminuria experienced a 21% (95% CI, 42%–0%; P = .0502) reduction in urine ACR, compared with placebo, whereas those starting with macroalbuminuria reduced their urine ACR by 39% on lixisenatide. Those without albuminuria did not experience significant reductions in urine ACR.

It is worth noting that GLP-1RA effects in reducing albuminuria and slowing eGFR decline do not prove that the class is renoprotective. Reductions in albuminuria are often associated with improved renal outcomes; however, changes to the eGFR trajectory seen with GLP-1RAs are less straightforward. Although SGLT-2i cause reduced albuminuria along with a decreased eGFR that remains stable, GLP-1RA do not affect renal hemodynamics and, in certain cases, have been shown to increase GFR. Such an increase was seen in AWARD-7 patients with macroalbuminuria taking dulaglutide and in LEADER participants with moderate or severe renal impairment taking liraglutide. A higher eGFR has the potential to increase glomerular pressure and thus speed renal decline. However, when compared with the placebo group, the rate of eGFR decline in the treatment group seems to be unaffected by GLP-1RA, and patients with CKD did not experience higher rates of adverse renal events.

Although individual GLP-1RA may differ, the class's ability to reduce urinary albumin excretions has larger health implications. An August 2019 meta-analysis across all relevant trials and publications found that the GLP-1RA class as a whole is associated with a 17% reduction to a composite kidney outcome composed of new-onset macroalbuminuria, decreased eGFR to creatinine ratio, ESKD, or death from renal causes.[30]

There is much left to learn about the GLP-1RA class's implications on the future standard of care for diabetic kidney disease. With the recent approval of the first oral form of GLP-1RA (oral semaglutide), investigation is also needed to elucidate whether the means of administration has any impact of renal protection or tolerance.[27]

SGLT-2i, the most recently developed class of oral medications in the type 2 diabetes landscape, work to lower HbA_{1c} and blood glucose by preventing glucose reabsorption in the proximal convoluted tubule. They are also associated with decreased blood pressure in part because of weight loss, natriuresis, and diuresis.[31] SGLT-2i are metabolized by the liver and the kidneys in varying degrees, depending on the individual drug. Thus, for those with liver or renal impairments, certain therapies may prove more tolerable than others. Because the presence of CKD affects the pharmacokinetic profile of the drug, a patient's renal status must be taken into account before prescribing SGLT-2i. For patients with mild CKD (eGFR 60–89 mL/min/1.73 m^2), no dose adjustment must be made. For patients with moderate CKD (eGFR 30–59 mL/min/1.73 m^2), SGLT-2i may be inappropriate, and if used, should be prescribed at a lower dosage. For patients with severe CKD (eGFR 15–29 mL/min/1.73 m^2), renal impairment, ESRD, or those on dialysis, SGLT-2i are currently contraindicated. The EMPA-REG OUTCOME trial and the CANVAS trial were two CV outcome trials whose renal outcomes suggest that SGLT-2i may confer renoprotective benefits.[32]

Empagliflozin was the third SGLT-2i to be approved by the Food and Drug Administration in 2014. Results from its CV outcome trial, EMPA-REG OUTCOME, contain data from primary CV end points and secondary renal microvascular outcomes. For 3.1 years, this randomized study followed 7020 patients with type 2 diabetes who had established CV disease and a glomerular filtration rate of greater than 30 mL/min/1.73 m^2 body surface area. In addition to their standard care, study participants took either 10-mg empagliflozin, 25-mg empagliflozin, or a placebo once a day. This study was the first to demonstrate that a glucose-lowering agent could also reduce the risk for major adverse CV events and heart failure hospitalizations, CV mortality, and overall mortality. But, the study's implications for renal protection also proved to be significant.[33]

The EMPA-REG OUTCOME trial used multiple renal outcomes to determine the long-term effects of empagliflozin on the kidney and on the progression of kidney disease. The first renal outcome was incident or worsening nephropathy. The study also used a composite outcome determined by incident or worsening nephropathy or CV death. Nephropathy was defined by multiple microvascular or clinically relevant outcomes that were also analyzed individually. These outcomes included: progression to macroalbuminuria, renal-replacement therapy initiation, doubling of serum creatinine level (eGFR ≤45 mL/min/1.73 m^2), and death caused by renal disease. Finally, the outcome of incident albuminuria in patients with normal baseline albumin levels was studied.[33]

Results of the study showed a significant 39% relative risk reduction in the incidence or worsening of nephropathy in the empagliflozin group (12.7%) compared with the placebo group (18.8%). Similarly, incident or worsening nephropathy or CV death was significantly reduced in the group receiving empagliflozin. Among the nephropathy outcomes, almost all showed significance. Progression to macroalbuminuria showed a significant relative risk reduction (38%) in the empagliflozin group (11.2%) compared with placebo (16.2%). Initiation of renal-replacement therapy had a 55% relative risk reduction for those on the empagliflozin therapy (0.3%) compared with those on placebo (0.6%). Empagliflozin led to a significant 44% relative risk reduction in serum creatinine level doubling (1.5% for empagliflozin and 2.6% for placebo). The rate of incident albuminuria and renal disease death did not show significant differences between groups.[33]

Empagliflozin was associated with higher rates of genital infections and urosepsis. However, the two groups were similar in rates of urinary tract infection, complicated urinary tract infection, pyelonephritis, diabetic ketoacidosis, hypoglycemic episodes, bone fractures, thromboembolic events, and events consistent with volume depletion. Patients on empagliflozin were also less likely to report events associated with acute kidney failure (hyperkalemia, acute kidney injury) compared with placebo.[33]

These findings prove promising for empagliflozin's renal protective effects. However, the results of this study may not be generalizable to all patient groups, particularly black patients (because of their small sample size) and type 2 patients with lower CV risk, because they were not included in the study. For type 2 patients with a high risk of CV events, the addition of empagliflozin to a standard care regimen was associated with a slower progression of CKD and a reduced risk for other adverse renal events.[33] The DECLARE-TIMI 58 (Dapagliflozin Effect on Cardiovascular Events–Thrombolysis in Myocardial Infarction 58) was the largest CV outcome trial to date for the SGLT-2i class, with 17,160 study participants with established CV disease or considered high risk. With regard to renal outcomes, the study showed a reduction in the secondary composite end point, composed of greater than or equal to 40% decrease in eGFR to less than 60 mL/min/1.73 m^2, new ESRD, or death from renal or CV cause (4.3% dapagliflozin and 5.6% placebo; HR, 0.76; 95% CI, 0.67–0.87). The treatment group also showed reductions in stabilized greater than or equal to 40% decrease in eGFR (to eGFR <60 mL/min/1.73 m^2), ESRD, or death from a renal cause, when compared with the placebo (1.5% and 2.8%, respectively; HR, 0.53; 95% CI, 0.43–0.66).[34]

The CANVAS program (composed of CANVAS and CANVAS Renal Endpoints) was a randomized, placebo-controlled trial studying canagliflozin in 10,142 type 2 patients with high CV risk for a median of 2.4 years. Although this trial associated canagliflozin treatment with increased risk of amputation and potential increased risk of bone fracture, study findings also showed canagliflozin's renoprotective effects, compared with placebo. These effects included reductions in the occurrence of albuminuria, the reduced likelihood of microalbuminuria or macroalbuminuria, and a slowed eGFR decline over time. Canagliflozin was also associated with a reduction in the frequency of a composite renal outcome that included persistent serum creatinine doubling, death caused by renal problems, and ESRD. Frequency of such renal outcomes in the treatment group compared with placebo was 1.5 versus 2.8 per 1000 patient-years, respectively (HR, 0.53; 95% CI, 0.33–0.84).[35] Post hoc analysis of CANVAS program data suggests that these effects are independent of baseline renal function in type 2 patients with high CV risk higher than eGFR levels of 30 mL/min/1.73 m^2. This finding holds potential for canagliflozin's use among patients whose eGFR levels fall lower than currently recommended levels.[32]

Unlike the SGLT-2i CV outcome trials, the CREDENCE (Canagliflozin and Renal Events in Diabetes with Established Nephropathy Clinical Evaluation) trial's primary objective was to study canagliflozin's effect on major renal outcomes in those considered at high risk for renal failure.[36]

CREDENCE studied canagliflozin in 4401 patients with type 2 diabetes and albuminuric CKD for a median of 2.62 years. Albuminuric CKD was defined as an eGFR of 30 to less than 90 mL/min/1.73 m^2 of body surface area and ACR ratio greater than 300 to 5000 mg/g. The randomized study compared the treatment group receiving 100-mg canagliflozin daily with placebo. All study participants were being treated with a renin-angiotensin system blocker. The trial's primary outcome was a renal composite consisting of doubling of serum creatinine levels, death from renal or CV causes, or ESKD. This study defined ESKD as the need for dialysis, renal transplant, or a consistent eGFR of less than 15 mL/min/1.73 m^2. Following a data and safety planning committee recommendation, the CREDENCE trial ended prematurely after preliminary results showed clear evidence of benefit for primary outcome measures ($P < .01$) and the composite outcome, which included ESKD or death from renal or CV causes.[36]

The CREDENCE study found a 30% lower relative risk for the renal composite primary outcome for those taking canagliflozin when compared with placebo. For this composite outcome, event rates were 43.2 per 1000 patient-years in those taking canagliflozin, compared with 61.2 for those on placebo (HR, 0.70; 95% CI, 0.59–0.82; $P = .00001$).

These results were consistent across CKD level subgroups. Canagliflozin was also associated with reduced risk for the individual components of the renal composite outcome, including occurrence of dialysis, kidney transplantation, or renal death (HR, 0.68; 95% CI, 0.54–0.86; P = .002) and serum creatinine level doubling (HR, 0.60; 95% CI, 0.48–0.76; P < .001). A secondary composite outcome included ESRD, doubling of serum creatinine level, or renal death. This secondary outcome had a relative risk reduction of 34% in the canagliflozin group. Rates of diabetic ketoacidosis were higher in the canagliflozin group than the placebo group (2.2 vs. 0.2 per 1000 patient-years), but unlike CANVAS results, amputation and bone fracture rates were not significantly different between the two groups. Although the treatment and placebo groups were similar in blood glucose level, blood pressure, and weight, the treatment group experienced reduced risk for the primary outcome and ESRD. This indicates that SGLT-2i benefit is the product of a mechanism beyond solely glucose level.[36]

At the time of the study, only renin-angiotensin system blockers were indicated as renoprotective drugs for those on a type 2 medication. Based on CREDENCE data, it is estimated that for every 1000 patients taking canagliflozin, 47 fewer would experience the primary composite outcome of ESKD, serum creatinine level doubling, or renal or CV death. However, it must be noted that this trial was stopped before reaching its planned number of events.[36] As eGFR decreases, so too does the effectiveness of SGLT-2i in improving blood glucose levels. However, SGLT-2i's renal and cardioprotective effects do not experience this same decline. These benefits persist across all eGFR levels greater than 30 mL/min/1.73 m². Although treatment with GLP-1RA does not alter the slope of the eGFR curve, CREDENCE findings show that SGLT-2i are capable of this effect.[27,36] For type 2 patients with CKD, SGLT-2i may further extend renal functioning and prevent the progression of renal disease (**Fig. 3**).

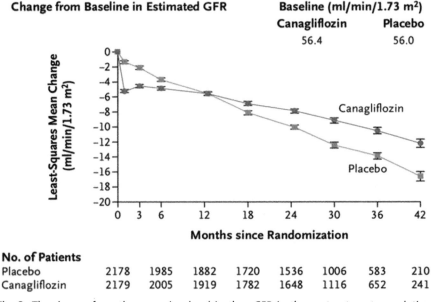

No. of Patients								
Placebo	2178	1985	1882	1720	1536	1006	583	210
Canagliflozin	2179	2005	1919	1782	1648	1116	652	241

Fig. 3. The change from the screening level in the eGFR in the on-treatment population. (*From* Perkovic V, Jardine MJ, Neal B, et al. Canagliflozin and renal outcomes in type 2 diabetes and nephropathy. N Engl J Med. 2019;380(24):2304; with permission.)

The benefits and risks that SGLT-2i confer seem to be consistent across the drug class. In addition to current standards of care, these drugs prove promising for not only glycemic control but also renoprotection.[37] A meta-analysis of the major CV outcome trials with renal data showed that treatment with SGLT-2i protects against acute renal injury and decreases risk of renal transplant, dialysis, or death because of renal disease.[38]

There is much left to be learned about the renal effects of GLP-1RA and SGLT-2i, with multiple clinical trials still underway. However, the renoprotective benefits already exhibited by these classes are promising, and their differing pharmacokinetic profiles leave open the possibility of future applications and perhaps combinations of these drugs.

DISCLOSURE

The authors have nothing to disclose.

REFERENCES

1. Krolewski AS, Warram JH, Christlieb AR, et al. The changing natural history of nephropathy in type I diabetes. Am J Med 1985;78(5):785–94.
2. Haneda M, Utsunomiya K, Koya D, et al. Shide K and Joint committee on Diabetic Nephropathy: a new classification of diabetic nephropathy 2014: a report from joint committee on diabetic nephropathy. J Diabetes Investig 2015;6(2):242–6.
3. KDIGO 2012. clinical practice guideline for the evaluation and management of chronic kidney disease. Kidney International Supplements 2013;3(1):1–150.
4. National Kidney Foundation. Summary of the MDRD study and CKD-EPI estimating equations. Available at: https://www.kidney.org/sites/default/files/docs/mdrd-study-and-ckd-epi-gfr-estimating-equations-summary-ta.pdf. Accessed May 7, 2020.
5. Stevens PE, Levin A. Kidney disease: improving global outcomes chronic kidney disease guideline development work group members: evaluation and management of chronic kidney disease: synopsis of the kidney disease: improving global outcomes 2012 clinical practice guideline. Ann Intern Med 2013;158(11):825–30.
6. Hommos MS, Glassock RJ, Rule AD. Structural and functional changes in human kidneys with healthy aging. J Am Soc Nephrol 2017;28(10):2838–44.
7. O'Sullivan ED, Hughes J, Ferenbach DA. Renal aging: causes and consequences. J Am Soc Nephrol 2017;28(2):407–20.
8. Gekle M. Kidney and aging: a narrative review. Exp Gerontol 2017;87(Pt B): 153–5.
9. Roseman DA, Hwang SJ, Oyama-Manabe N, et al. Clinical associations of total kidney volume: the Framingham Heart Study. Nephrol Dial Transplant 2017; 32(8):1344–50.
10. Wang X, Vrtiska TJ, Avula RT, et al. Age, kidney function, and risk factors associate differently with cortical and medullary volumes of the kidney. Kidney Int 2014;85(3):677–85.
11. Rule AD, Sasiwimonphan K, Lieske JC, et al. Characteristics of renal cystic and solid lesions based on contrast enhanced computed tomography of potential kidney donors. Am J Kidney Dis 2012;59(5):611–8.
12. Abdelhafiz AH, Nahas ME, de Oliveira JM. Management of diabetic nephropathy in older patients: a need for flexible guidelines. Postgrad Med 2014;126(4): 171–7.

13. American Diabetes Association. Microvascular complications and foot care: standards of medical care in diabetes—2019. Diabetes Care 2019;42(Supplement 1): S124–9.

14. National Kidney Foundation. KDOQI clinical practice guideline for diabetes and CKD: 2012 update. Am J Kidney Dis 2012;60(5):850–86.

15. Pavkov ME, Collins AJ, Josef Coresh J, et al. Kidney disease in diabetes. In: Cowie CC, Casagrande SS, Menke A, et al, editors. Chapter 22 in Diabetes in America. 3rd edition. Bethesda (MD): National Institutes of Health, NIH Pub No. 17-1468; 2018. p. 22-1–22-84. Available at: https://www.niddk.nih.gov/-/media/Files/Strategic-Plans/Diabetes-in-America-3rd-Edition/DIA_Ch22.pdf?la=en&hash=B36A992469526A5C4C240263AB81E0BC.

16. Mann JF, Schmieder RE, McQueen M, et al. Renal outcomes with telmisartan, ramipril, or both, in people at high vascular risk (the ONTARGET study): a multicentre, randomised, double-blind, controlled trial. The Lancet 2008;372(9638): 547–53.

17. Van Hateren KJ, Landman GW, Kleefstra N, et al. Lower blood pressure associated with higher mortality in elderly diabetic patients (ZODIAC-12). Age Ageing 2010;39(5):603–9.

18. Gerstein HC, Miller ME, Byrington RP. Action to control cardiovascular risk in diabetes study group. Effects of intensive glucose lowering in type 2 diabetes. N Engl J Med 2008;358(24):2545–59.

19. Cooper-DeHoff RM, Gong Y, Handberg EM, et al. Tight blood pressure control and cardiovascular outcomes among hypertensive patients with diabetes and coronary artery disease. JAMA 2010;304(1):61–8.

20. Petersen LK, Christensen K, Kragstrup J. Lipid-lowering treatment to the end? A review of observational studies and RCTs on cholesterol and mortality in 80+ year olds. Age Ageing 2010;39(6):674–80.

21. Nadolnik K, Skrypnik D, Skypnik K, et al. Diabetic nephropathy in the elderly-clinical practice. Rocz Panstw Zaki Hig 2018;69(4):327–34.

22. Kramer H, Boucher RE, Leehey D, et al. Increasing mortality in adults with diabetes and low estimated glomerular filtration rate in the absence of albuminuria. Diabetes Care 2018;41(4):775–81.

23. Vistisen D, Andersen GS, Hulman A, et al. Progressive decline in estimated glomerular filtration rate in patients with diabetes after moderate loss in kidney function—even without albuminuria. Diabetes Care 2019;42(10):1886–94.

24. Penno G, Solini A, Orsi E, et al, Renal Insufficiency and Cardiovascular Events (RIACE) Study Group. Non-albuminuric renal impairment is a strong predictor of mortality in individuals with type 2 diabetes: the Renal Insufficiency and Cardiovascular Events (RIACE) Italian multicentre study. Diabetologia 2018;61(11): 2277–89.

25. Anyanwagu U, Donnelly R, Idris I. Individual and combined relationship between reduced eGFR and/or increased urinary albumin excretion rate with mortality risk among insulin-treated patients with type 2 diabetes in routine practice. Kidney Dis (Basel) 2019;5(2):91–9.

26. Giugliano D, De Nicola L, Maiorino MI, et al. Type 2 diabetes and the kidney: insights from cardiovascular outcome trials. Diabetes Obes Metab 2019;21(8): 1790–800.

27. van Baar MJB, van der Aart AB, Hoogenberg K, et al. The incretin pathway as a therapeutic target in diabetic kidney disease: a clinical focus on GLP-1 receptor agonists. Ther Adv Endocrinol Metab 2019;10: 2042018819865398.

28. Mann JFE, Ørsted DD, Brown-Frandsen K, et al. LEADER steering committee and investigators. liraglutide and renal outcomes in type 2 diabetes. N Engl J Med 2017;377(9):839–48.
29. Marso SP, Bain SC, Consoli A, et al, SUSTAIN-6 Investigators. Semaglutide and cardiovascular outcomes in patients with type 2 diabetes. N Engl J Med 2016; 375(19):1834–44.
30. Kristensen SL, Rørth R, Jhund PS, et al. Cardiovascular, mortality, and kidney outcomes with GLP-1 receptor agonists in patients with type 2 diabetes: a systematic review and meta-analysis of cardiovascular outcome trials. Lancet Diabetes Endocrinol 2019;7(10):776–85.
31. de Albuquerque Rocha N, Neeland IJ, McCullough PA, et al. Effects of sodium glucose co-transporter 2 inhibitors on the kidney. Diab Vasc Dis Res 2018; 15(5):375–86.
32. Davidson JA. SGLT2 inhibitors in patients with type 2 diabetes and renal disease: overview of current evidence. Postgrad Med 2019;131(4):251–60.
33. Wanner C, Inzucchi SE, Lachin JM, et al, EMPA-REG OUTCOME Investigators. Empagliflozin and progression of kidney disease in type 2 diabetes. N Engl J Med 2016;375(4):323–34.
34. Mosenzon O, Wiviott SD, Cahn A, et al. Effects of dapagliflozin on development and progression of kidney disease in patients with type 2 diabetes: an analysis from the DECLARE-TIMI 58 randomised trial. Lancet Diabetes Endocrinol 2019; 7(8):606–17.
35. Neal B, Perkovic V, Mahaffey KW, et al, CANVAS Program Collaborative Group. Canagliflozin and cardiovascular and renal events in type 2 diabetes. N Engl J Med 2017;377(7):644–57.
36. Perkovic V, Jardine MJ, Neal B, et al, CREDENCE Trial Investigators. Canagliflozin and renal outcomes in type 2 diabetes and nephropathy. N Engl J Med 2019; 380(24):2295–306.
37. van Bommel EJ, Muskiet MH, Tonneijck L, et al. SGLT2 inhibition in the diabetic kidney-from mechanisms to clinical outcome. Clin J Am Soc Nephrol 2017; 12(4):700–10.
38. Neuen BL, Young T, Heerspink HJL, et al. SGLT2 inhibitors for the prevention of kidney failure in patients with type 2 diabetes: a systematic review and meta-analysis. Lancet Diabetes Endocrinol 2019;7(11):845–54.

Diabetes and Heart Failure
A Marriage of Inconvenience

Adi Mehta, MD, FRCPC[a],*, Sanjeeb Bhattacharya, MD[b],
Jerry Estep, MD[b], Charles Faiman, MD, FRCPC, MACE[c]

KEYWORDS

• Diabetes • Heart failure • Hyperglycemia • Diabetic cardiomyopathy

KEY POINTS

• Type 2 diabetes and heart failure are increasingly becoming a public health crisis associated with a rising prevalence and staggering health care costs.
• Ongoing research has shown a distinct etiopathophysiologic link between type 2 diabetes and the development of cardiomyopathy.
• Until recently, diabetes and heart failure treatments were geared to treating the 2 distinct disease processes with concerns regarding the effect of each treatment program on the alternate disease process. Currently, newer medical therapies target both disease processes simultaneously, thereby improving both diabetes and cardiovascular outcomes.

Type 2 diabetes has become a national and global epidemic, which history will likely designate as the plague of the early twenty-first century. It is expected that nearly 600 million individuals will be affected worldwide within the next 15 years, constituting a doubling from 2010 to 2035.[1] In the United States, statistics from the American Diabetes Association reported a prevalence of 9.4%, or about 30.3 million individuals of which 7.2 million or 25% were undiagnosed. The prevalence in the over 65 age group was significantly higher at 25.2% or 2 million individuals. Moreover, it was estimated that 84.1 million persons in the over 18 age group had prediabetes.[2] All of the above estimates are expected to increase exponentially within the next 15 to 20 years.

Heart failure (HF) has also become a major public health crisis. It is estimated that more than 5.7 million people in the United States suffer from congestive HF , a number slated to increase.[3] The health care costs are estimated to be more than a staggering 30 billion dollars per year. It is expected that the number of individuals with HF in the

[a] Endocrinology and Metabolism Institute, Cleveland Clinic, 9500 Euclid Avenue, F-20, Cleveland, OH 44195, USA; [b] Section of Heart Failure and Cardiac Transplant Medicine, Cleveland Clinic, 9500 Euclid Avenue, J3-4, Cleveland, OH 44195, USA; [c] Department of Endocrinology, Cleveland Clinic, 9500 Euclid Avenue, F-20, Cleveland, OH 44195, USA
* Corresponding author.
E-mail address: mehtaae@ccf.org
Twitter: @SBhattacharyaMD (S.B.)

Clin Geriatr Med 36 (2020) 447–455
https://doi.org/10.1016/j.cger.2020.04.005
0749-0690/20/© 2020 Elsevier Inc. All rights reserved.
geriatric.theclinics.com

United States will double between the years 2000 and 2035.[4] Just as in diabetes, the prevalence of HF is 3-fold higher in the over 60 age group.

HF is categorized based on left ventricular ejection fraction (LVEF) defined by cardiac imaging. Heart failure with reduced ejection fraction (HFrEF) entails all cardiomyopathies with an ejection fraction less than 40%, with preserved ejection fraction (HFpEF) traditionally being greater than 40%. More recently, there has been a further delineation with mildly reduced ejection fraction (LVEF > 40% and <50%) and preserved ejection fraction (LVEF > 50%).[5] The groupings are important given the strength of guideline-directed therapy in the HFrEF population, whereas HFpEF has yet to find any therapies to improve survival.

There are a large number of epidemiologic studies evaluating the relationship of HF and diabetes; the Framingham Heart Study exemplifies this relationship between diabetes and HF: HF is twice as frequent in men and nearly 5 times more frequent in women with diabetes as in a nondiabetes population.[6] Conversely, the overall prevalence of diabetes in patients with HF has been reported to be as high as 44% compared with the circa 10% prevalence of diabetes in the general population.[7] Although there is an increased prevalence of the metabolic syndrome, characterized by the presence of abdominal obesity, hypertension, atherogenic dyslipidemia, and dysglycemia in HF, the association of diabetes, itself, with HF persists after adjusting for these metabolic syndrome factors, suggesting an independent cause-and-effect relationship.[8]

THE PATHOPHYSIOLOGY OF HEART FAILURE IN DIABETES

The physiology in diabetic cardiomyopathies is complex. There is an important relationship between insulin resistance (IR) and HF. IR is an independent predictor of HF. Ingelsson and colleagues[9] showed that in a 9-year follow-up study of more than 12,000 men over the age of 70, the incidence of HF increased from 5 per 1000 person-years in the most insulin-sensitive quartile to 16 per 1000 person-years in the most insulin-resistant quartile.

It is well described that in the normal heart, healthy cardiomyocytes use free fatty acids (FFA) as the primary source of fuel with low reliance on glucose metabolism, particularly during exercise when glucose and pyruvate oxidation become increasingly impaired.[10] With IR, there is increased lipolysis in adipose tissue releasing elevated levels of FFA into the circulation. The excess FFA associated with a concomitant decrease in glucose transport into the cell, because of IR-associated depletion of GLUT-1 and -4 receptors, results in excess FFA transport into the cardiomyocyte. FFA metabolism requires high oxygen consumption so that any decrease in oxygen supply impairs FFA metabolism, causing intracellular FFA accumulation leading to excess intracellular triglyceride.[10–12] McGavock and colleagues[13] found that in myocardial biopsy specimens from more than 130 individuals, intramyocardial triglyceride increased from 0.46% fat/water ratio in lean individuals, to 0.81% fat/water ratio in obese normoglycemic individuals, to 0.95% in individuals with impaired glucose tolerance and 1.06% in individuals with type 2 diabetes, suggesting that IR, present even before glucose abnormalities, was associated with significant histologic cardiomyocyte lipid accumulation.

The increase in intracellular FFA also induces adverse effects on the structure and function of the cardiomyocyte. Structurally, high intracellular FFA compromises the mitochondrial respiratory chain, generating reactive oxygen species (ROS) and ceramides. Increased ROS damages and modifies cellular structural proteins, resulting in cellular damage, apoptosis, and necrosis, initiating a chronic inflammatory state, leading to functional impairment. Such a cascade of events promotes remodeling of collagen tissue and results in fibrosis, compounding cardiac dysfunction.[12,14] Thus, this deranged myocardial metabolism ultimately leads to impaired myocardial relaxation and contractility. ROS further worsens IR, setting up a vicious cycle.[12]

With the progressive worsening of IR, the compensatory reserve of the β cell becomes increasingly compromised, resulting in worsening hyperglycemia. High glucose and more importantly the greater excursions in circulating glucose values acutely impair endothelium-dependent vasodilatation by inhibiting nitric oxide generation. Such vasoconstriction further decreases oxidative metabolism and initiates the deleterious cycle of further intracellular FFA and triglyceride accumulation[15,16]

Established hyperglycemia predisposes to increased protein glycation, and the accumulation of advanced glycation end products (AGEs), accumulation contributes to morphologic changes of cardiomyocytes. AGE accumulation changes the function of the proteins affected, resulting in decreased elasticity of both cardiomyocytes and vessel walls, leading to further impairment in cardiac mechanics. It has been shown that isovolumic relaxation time is prolonged in direct correlation to serum levels of AGEs.[17]

These alterations in cardiomyocyte metabolism and sequelae cause distinct alterations in cardiac structure and mechanics as well as endothelial function in diabetic cardiomyopathies. Myocardial hypertrophy and fibrosis lead to abnormalities in diastology, presenting more of a restrictive or HFpEF phenotype, whereas increased oxidative stress leading to increased apoptosis can ultimately lead to a dilated cardiomyopathy or HFrEF phenotype.[18]

Therapeutic Implications for Patients with Diabetes and Heart Failure

Given the pathophysiology outlined above, prevention of HF is almost synonymous with preventing type 2 diabetes and decreasing IR. Previously, diabetic therapy was directed at controlling hyperglycemia that would not aggravate fluid retention and had minimal cardiac toxicity. Currently, newer medications directed at diabetes management have been shown to have profound beneficial effects in HF management.

Effects of Diabetes-Related Therapies Effect on Heart Failure

Glucose control

There is a complicated relationship between glucose control and HF. In a Swedish study with a follow-up of more than 83,000 patients, after adjusting for known risk factors for HF, for each 1% increase in hemoglobin A1c (HbA1c), there was a 12% increase in hospitalization for HF.[19] Interestingly, there have not been data to show strict glycemic control leading to reducing incidence of HF in patients with diabetes. A metaanalysis of data from more than 37,000 patients in 3 major intensive control of hyperglycemia trials (ACCORD, ADVANCE, and VADT) failed to show a favorable effect of intensive glucose control on preventing HF.[20] In fact, in another study of almost 9000 patients with diabetes (GoDarts study), although poor glycemic control was associated with a higher risk for HF (HbA1c > 6.9% was associated with a 2.26-fold increase in HF risk), more surprisingly, intensive glucose control with HbA1c averaging less than 6% also had an increased risk of chronic HF (odds ratio 2.48). Thus, the control of glucose seems to have a minimal effect on HF; it is more likely that the modalities used to treat the hyperglycemia play a more important role on HF independent of their glucose effect.

Effects of Glucose-Related Interventions on Heart Failure

Diet and exercise

Healthy diet and exercise are routinely recommended to promote weight loss in diabetes because numerous well-done studies have consistently shown benefit in terms of short-term and long-term outcomes with regards to prevention of diabetes and control of established hyperglycemia. Diet and exercise are also recommended early in HF. However, there are no good prospective trials that show benefit. The Look AHEAD study in 5145 obese patients with type 2 diabetes showed no significant effect on HF despite improved fitness, glucose control, and some weight loss. Larger amounts of weight loss following bariatric surgery have shown a decreased incidence of HF. However, studies in patients on DASH or Mediterranean diets have shown inconsistent benefits on diastolic and systolic function in patients with HF. The bottom line, as outlined in the American College of Cardiology Nutrition and Lifestyle Committee report on the prevention of cardiovascular (CV) disease, is that it cannot be recommended that maintenance of normal weight throughout life would be protective against HF. Moreover, sodium restriction even in established HF has yet to be of proven benefit. Nonetheless, cardiorespiratory fitness has been directly related to a decreased incidence of HF, and exercise therapy to increase cardiorespiratory fitness has been shown to have functional benefits in HF. In much smaller studies, yoga and transcendental meditation have shown some degree of symptomatic benefits in advanced HF, but there are no large randomized controlled trials to prove or disprove the point.[21]

Older Traditional Antihyperglycemic Agents

Metformin
Metformin is universally accepted as the first-line therapy in the pharmaceutical treatment of type 2 diabetes. It has been used alone or in combination with every other class of antihyperglycemic agents. With specific regards to HF in patients with diabetes, metformin, which was originally relatively contraindicated in HF for fear of an increased lactic acidosis potential, has been associated with better short-term and long-term prognosis and reduced incidence of HF hospitalizations and reduced mortality in patients with HF or with chronic kidney disease, according to a recent metaanalysis.[22] However, another metaanalysis of randomized metformin intervention trials failed to show a reduction in HF.[23] Metformin has been shown to reduce cardiac hypertrophy by an as-yet undefined mechanism. One proposed mechanism is repressing mammalian target of rapamycin (mTOR) activity by increasing mitochondrial 5' adenosine monophosphate-activated protein kinase (AMPK), thereby reducing abnormal protein synthesis and stimulating glucose uptake.

Sulfonylureas
These agents are the old standby for treating type 2 diabetes. With the advent of newer agents less likely to cause hypoglycemia and weight gain, use of sulfonylureas (SFU) has fallen into disfavor, but because of their significantly lower cost, the frequency of utilization is higher than most guidelines would recommend. The association of SFU and HF has been underappreciated and therefore underestimated and underreported. SFUs can induce weight gain, which can increase the risk of HF by 7.1% per each kilogram increase.[24] Furthermore, in the UK General Practice database analysis, SFU use was associated with an 18% to 30% increased risk of HF.[25] Similarly, in the Veterans Health Administration database, SFU use was associated with a 32% increase in HF.[26] A metaanalysis of observational studies showed an aggregate risk of 17% to 22% in HF in patients on SFU, and the risk was dose dependent.[27] As well, SFU use in patients with coexisting diabetes and HF is associated with an increased risk of death.[28]

Thiazolidinediones
These agents were highly anticipated for glycemic control as well as for the potential benefits for HF. In in vitro and in vivo animal studies, thiazolidinediones (TZDs) are able to significantly alter FFA metabolism by redirecting the FFA into preadipocytes,

thereby limiting their availability as an alternative fuel, thus, reducing intracellular triglyceride accumulation in cardiomyocytes in rats. However, this perceived benefit did not translate clinically as TZDs led to worsening heart failure outcomes. In the Pro-Active study, the largest study with pioglitazone, there was a higher incidence of HF (5.7% in the pioglitazone group and 4.1% in the placebo group).[29] Thus, TZDs have been contraindicated in patients with HF.

Newer Antihyperglycemic Agents

Glucagon-like peptide-1 agonists
These agents are emerging as cardioprotective in diabetes, having shown a significant reduction in MACE (multivariate analysis of CV events) encompassing CV death, nonfatal myocardial infarction (MI), and nonfatal stroke. In the CardioVascular Outcome Trials (CVOT) studies of these agents, there has been no signal for an effect on HF.[30] In small preclinical studies, native glucagon-like peptide-1 (GLP-1), when infused in acute MI, showed improvement in wall motion and ejection fraction.[31]

Dipeptidyl peptidase-4 inhibitors
Experimental studies in animals and humans with dipeptidyl peptidase-4 (DPP-4) inhibitors have shown improvement in cardiac function probably because of the enhanced endogenous GLP-1 level induced by the blockade of the DPP-4 enzyme. In clinical practice, all of the US-licensed DPP-4 inhibitors that have completed CVOT trials seem to be cardioneutral, whereas data-mining studies of real-world use show some CV benefit. Only 1 agent, saxagliptin, showed a significantly increased incidence of HF in the Savor-Timi53 trial.[32] The CVOTs of the other drugs in the class individually were neutral with regards to HF, but a metaanalysis of studies of these drugs, including data from the CVOTs, suggested a small increase in hospitalizations for HF.[33] However, there are no black box warnings with regards to HF for these agents, except saxagliptin, and the consensus seems to be to continue these agents in compensated and controlled HF using clinical judgment.

Sodium glucose co-transporter-2 inhibitors
These agents have made a significant impact on the treatment of HF in diabetes. The enhanced glycosuric effect of these agents is accompanied by natriuresis. Although this clearly has the same effect as diuretics, there seems to be a more salutary sodium preservation effect intracellularly, which tends to preserve and enhance cardiomyocyte integrity and improve diastolic function (now being studied in the EMPERIAL-PRESERVED trial). All CVOT studies with these agents have shown a substantial beneficial effect on HF reducing hospitalization for HF by 21%.[34–37] Recently, a study in individuals with HF showed benefits of these agents in HF even in those without diabetes.[38] There are numerous hypothesized potential proposed mechanisms for this benefit: increased natriuresis; a higher hematocrit seen in the blood count panel; a decrease in blood pressure; the renal protection induced by the decrease in renal work load; the possible beneficial effect of the increase in circulating ketones which, in the presence of circulating insulin, serve as another cellular fuel source competing successfully with FFA for myocardial energy generation; the less appreciated decrease in IR induced by these agents; and, of course, the weight loss induced by these agents.[39]

Insulin
Insulin, aside from its effects on glucose, causes retention of sodium and water.[40] Some observational studies showed an increased risk of HF.[41] However, CVOTs using long-acting insulin analogues have not shown an increase in CV risk or HF risk.[42–44]

Short-acting insulins have no CVOTs to date, but studies documenting their efficacy had no adverse HF signals.[45]

Traditional Heart Failure Therapies and Effect on Diabetic Control

HF has been thoroughly and thoughtfully studied over the last 30 years, and the results have brought us several classes of drugs that can be used to treat HF and particularly HFrEF. Although they have profound effects on CV outcomes, little attention is paid to their metabolic side effects.

Beta-blockers
Beta-blockers have been a mainstay of therapy in patients with HFreF with a profound effect on mortality and sudden cardiac death. The COPERNICUS study with carvedilol showed a marked reduction in mortality within the first 8 weeks of initiation. Three particular beta-blockers used in HFrEF for their mortality benefit are carvedilol, bisoprolol, and metoprolol. Beta-blockers have shown an adverse metabolic effect, resulting in an increase in HbA1c. When comparing metoprolol and carvedilol, metoprolol modestly increased HbA1c, whereas carvedilol seemed to improve insulin sensitivity.[46] It is important to note that beta-blockers can mask the symptoms of hypoglycemia, so, especially in the older adult treated with antidiabetes agents predisposing to hypoglycemia, beta-blocker therapy can add an enhanced level of risk.

Angiotensin-converting enzyme inhibitors and angiotensin receptor blockers
Both angiotensin-converting enzyme (ACE) inhibitors and angiotensin receptor blockers (ARB) have mortality benefit in the treatment of HFrEF. In addition, there are some data indicating that ARB can be beneficial in HFpEF when looking at HF hospitalization. Both classes have been shown not to increase the risk of diabetes and may have some protective effects. In the HOPE trial, the use of ramipril showed a reduction in the development of diabetes. Candesartan showed a similar metabolic profile in the CHARM trial.[47]

Mineralocorticoid receptor antagonist
The additive effects of mineralocorticoid receptor antagonist (MRA) in reducing mortality and sudden cardiac death on the backbone of beta-blocker and ACE have been shown in multiple studies. Spironolactone has been shown to worsen glycemic control and increase HbA1c levels by 0.2%, whereas eplerenone did not show a similar metabolic side effect.[48]

Neprolysin inhibitor
Sacubatril-valsartan is a newer drug with profound effects on HFreF as well as a modest impact on HFpEF patients. PARADIGM was the largest trial in HFrEF patients and showed a significant mortality benefit when comparing sacubatril-valsartan to enalapril. In a post hoc analysis of PARADIGM, sacubatril-valsartan showed improved glycemic control when compared with enalapril. There was a reduction of 0.26% in HbA1c over 1 year and a 29% lower incidence of insulin use in the sacubatril-valsartan arm.[49]

SUMMARY

IR has a powerful pathophysiologic role altering intracellular fuel utilization and metabolism, thereby inducing a cascade of increased ROS, inflammation, and fibrosis leading to derangements of cardiac function and mechanics. This condition is further aggravated by the development of hyperglycemia when compensatory insulin capacity becomes impaired, resulting in increased production of AGEs, leading to further disruption of cardiomyocyte structure and function. Risk factors associated with diabetes, including hypertension, dyslipidemia, and coronary artery disease, amplify the cardiac dysfunction, further increasing the risk of HF. Until recently, there has been a separated approach to the treatment of diabetes and HF, concentrating specific drugs for the specific disease. Currently, there is a shift in perspective, studying agents that exert a dual benefit in glycemic and HF control or prevention. As these agents are pushed to the forefront, more data will be needed on risk/benefit utilization in the aging population.

DISCLOSURE

A. Mehta: speakers bureau: Novo-Nordisk, Boehringer-Ingelheim. The other authors have nothing to disclose.

REFERENCES

1. Guariguata L, Whiting DR, Hambleton I, et al. Global estimates of diabetes prevalence for 2013 and projections for 2035. Diabetes Res Clin Pract 2014;103: 137–49.
2. Zimmet P, Alberti KA, Magliano DJ, et al. Diabetes mellitus statistics on prevalence and mortality: facts and fallacies. Nat Rev Endocrinol 2016;12:616–22.
3. Mozzafarian D, Benjamin EJ, Go AS, et al, on behalf of the American Heart Association Statistics Committee and Stroke Statistics Subcommittee. Heart disease and stroke statistics—2016 update: a report from the American Heart Association. Circulation 2016;133:e38–360.
4. Dei Cas A, Khan SS, Butler J, et al. Impact of diabetes on epidemiology, treatment and outcomes of patients with heart failure. JACC Heart Fail 2015;3:136–45.
5. Alagiakrishnan K, Banach M, Jones LG, et al. Update on diastolic heart failure or heart failure with preserved ejection in the older adults. Ann Med 2013;45:37–50.
6. Kannel WB, McGee DL. Diabetes and cardiovascular disease. The Framingham study. JAMA 1979;241:2035–8.
7. Rubler S, Dlugash J, Yuceoglu YZ, et al. New type of cardiomyopathy associated ith diabetic glomerulosclerosis. Am J Cardiol 1972;30:595–602.
8. Echouffo-Tcheugui JB, Xu H, Devore AD, et al. Temporal trends and factors associated with diabetes mellitus among patients hospitalized with heart failure; findings from Get With The Guidelines–Heart Failure registry. Am Heart J 2016; 182:9–20.
9. Ingelsson E, Sundstrom J, Arnlov J, et al. Insulin resistance and risk of congestive heart failure. JAMA 2005;294:334–42.
10. Neubauer S. The failing heart–an engine out of fuel. N Engl J Med 2007;356: 1140–51.
11. Russell RR III, Yin R, Caplan M, et al. Additive effects of hyperinsulinemia and ischemia on myocardial GLUT 1 and GLUT 4 translocation in vivo. Circulation 1998;98:2180–6.
12. Nishikawa T, Araki E. Impact of mitochondrial ROS production in the pathogenesis of diabetes mellitus and its complications. Antioxid Redox Signal 2007;9: 34–53.
13. McGavock JM, Lingvay I, Zib I, et al. Cardiac steatosis in diabetes mellitus: a 1H-magnetic resonance spectroscopy study. Circulation 2007;116:1170–5.
14. Heerebeek VL, Hamdani N, Handoko ML, et al. Diastolic stiffness of the failing diabetic heart. Importance of fibrosis, advanced glycation end products, and myocyte resting tension. Circulation 2008;117:43–51.

15. Kawano H, Motoyama T, Hirashima O, et al. Hyperglycemia rapidly suppresses flow mediated endothelium dependent vasodilatation of brachial artery. J Am Coll Cardiol 1999;34:146–54.

16. DiFlavian A, Picconi F, Di Stefano P, et al. Impact of glycemic and blood pressure variability on surrogate measures of cardiovascular outcomes in type 2 diabetic patients. Diabetes Care 2011;34:1605–9.

17. Goldin A, Beckman JA, Schmidt AM, et al. Advanced glycation end products: sparking the development of diabetic vascular injury. Circulation 2006;114:597–605.

18. Seferovic P, Paulus WJ. Clinical diabetic cardiomyopathy: a two-faced disease with restrictive and dilated phenotypes. Eur Heart J 2015;35:1718–27.

19. Lind M, Olsson M, Rosengren A, et al. The relationship between glycemic control and heart failure in 83021 patients with type 2 diabetes. Diabetologia 2012;55:2946–53.

20. Castagno D, Baird-Gunning J, Jhund PS, et al. Intensive glycemic control has no impact on the risk of heart failure in type 2 diabetes, evidence from a 37,229 patient meta-analysis. Am Heart J 2011;162:938–48.

21. Aggarwal M, Bozkurt B, Panjrath G, et al. Lifestyle modifications for preventing and treating heart failure. J Am Coll Cardiol 2018;72:2391–405.

22. Crowley MJ, Diamantidis CJ, McDuffie JR, et al. Clinical outcomes of metformin use in populations with chronic kidney disease, congestive heart failure or chronic liver disease: a systemic review. Ann Intern Med 2017;166:191–200.

23. Boussageon R, Supper I, Bejan-Angoulvant T, et al. Reappraisal of metformin efficacy in the treatment of type 2 diabetes: a meta-analysis of randomized controlled trials. PLoS Med 2012;9:e1001204.

24. Udell JA, Cavender MA, Bhatt DL, et al. Glucose-lowering drugs or strategies and cardiovascular outcomes in patients with or at risk for type 2 diabetes: a meta-analysis of randomized controlled trials. Lancet Diabetes Endocrinol 2015;3:356–66.

25. Tzoulaki I, Molokhia M, Curcin V, et al. Risk of cardiovascular disease and all cause mortality among patients with type 2 diabetes prescribed oral antidiabetes drugs: retrospective cohort study using UK general practice research database. BMJ 2009;339:b4731.

26. Roumie CL, Min JY, D'Agostino McGowan L, et al. Comparative safety of sulfonylurea and metformin monotherapy on the risk of heart failure: a cohort study. J Am Heart Assoc 2017;6:e005379.

27. Varas-Lorenzo C, Margulis A, Perez-Gutthann S, et al. The risk of heart failure associated with the use of noninsulin blood glucose-lowering drugs: systematic review and meta-analysis of published observational studies. BMC Cardiovasc Disord 2014;14:129.

28. McAlister FA, Eurich DT, Majumdar SR, et al. The risk of heart failure in patients with type 2 diabetes treated with oral agent monotherapy. Eur J Heart Fail 2008;10:703–8.

29. Dormandy J, Bhattacharya M, van Troostenburg de Bruyn AR, et al. Safety and tolerability of pioglitazone in high-risk patients with type 2 diabetes: an overview of data from PROactive trial. Drug Saf 2009;32:187–202.

30. Li L, Li S, Liu J, et al. Glucagon-like peptide-1 receptor agonists and heart failure in type 2 diabetes: systemic review and meta-analysis of randomized and observational studies. BMC Cardiovasc Disord 2016;16:91.

31. Sokos GG, Nikolaidis LA, Mankad S, et al. Glucagon-like peptide 1 infusion improves left ventricular ejection fraction and functional status in patients with chronic heart failure. J Card Fail 2006;12:694–9.
32. Scirica BM, Bhatt DL, Braunwald E, et al. Saxagliptin and cardiovascular outcomes in patients with type 2 diabetes mellitus. N Engl J Med 2013;369:1317–26.
33. Scheen AJ. Cardiovascular effects of new oral glucose lowering agents: DPP-4 and SGLT-2 inhibitors. Circ Res 2018;122:1439–59.
34. Zinman B, Wanner C, Lachin JM, et al. Empagliflozin, cardiovascular outcomes and mortality in type 2 diabetes. N Engl J Med 2015;373:2117–28.
35. Neal B, Perkovic V, Mahaffey K, et al. Canagliflozin and cardiovascular and renal events in type 2 diabetes. N Engl J Med 2017;377:644–57.
36. Sonesson C, Johansson PA, Johnsson E, et al. Cardiovascular effects of depagliflozin in patients with type 2 diabetes and different risk categories: a meta-analysis. Cardiovasc Diabetol 2016;15:37.
37. Wiviott SD, Raz I, Bonaca MP, et al. Dapagliflozin and cardiovascular outcomes in type 2 diabetes. N Engl J Med 2019;380:347–57.
38. McMurray JJV, Solomon SD, Inzucchi SE, et al. Dapagliflozin in patients with heart failure and reduced ejection fraction. N Engl J Med 2020;382(10):973.
39. Kaplan A, Abidi E, El-Yazbi A, et al. Direct cardiovascular impact of SGLT-2 inhibitor: mechanisms and effects. Heart Fail Rev 2018;23:419–37.
40. Nolan CJ, Ruderman NB, Kahn SE, et al. Intensive insulin for type 2 diabetes: the risk of causing harm. Lancet Diabetes Endocrinol 2013;1:9–10.
41. Hippislet-Coc J, Coupland C. Diabetes treatments and risk of heart failure, cardiovascular disease and all cause mortality: cohort study in primary care. BMJ 2016;354:3477.
42. Gerstein HC, Bosch HC, Dagenais GR, et al. Basal insulin and cardiovascular and other outcomes in dysglycemia. N Engl J Med 2012;367:319–28.
43. Gerstein HC, Jung H, Rydén L, et al. Effect of basal insulin glargine on first and recurrent episodes of heart failure hospitalizations: the ORIgiN trial. Circulation 2018;37:88–90.
44. Marso SP, McGuire Dk, Zinman B, et al. Efficacy and safety of degludec verses glargine in type 2 diabetes. N Engl J Med 2017;377:723–32.
45. Rathmann W, Schloot NC, Kostev K, et al. Macro- and microvascular outcomes in patients with type 2 diabetes treated with rapid-acting insulin analogues or human regular insulin: a retrospective database analysis. Exp Clin Endocrinol Diabetes 2014;122:92–9.
46. Bakris GL, Fonseca V, Katholi RE, et al. Metabolic effects of carvedilol vs metoprolol in patients with type2 diabetes mellitus and hypertension: a randomized controlled trial. JAMA 2004;292(18):2227–36.
47. Grodzinsky A, Arnold SV, Jacob D, et al. The impact of cardiovascular drugs on diabetes: a review. Endocr Pract 2017;23(3):363–71.
48. Yamaji M, Tsutamoto T, Kawahara C, et al. Effect of eplerenone versus spironolactone on cortisol and hemoglobin A(1)(c) levels in patients with chronic heart failure. Am Heart J 2010;160(5):915–21.
49. Seferovic J, Claggett B, Seidelmann SB, et al. Effect of sacubatril/valsartan versus enalapril on glycaemic control in patients with heart failure and diabetes: a post-hoc analysis from PARADIGM-HF trial. Lancet 2017;5(5):333–40.

Treating Dyslipidemias in the Primary Prevention of Atherosclerotic Cardiovascular Disease in Older Adults with Diabetes Mellitus

MengHee Tan, MD[a],*, Mark Paul MacEachern, MLIS[b]

KEYWORDS

- Older people with diabetes • Dyslipidemias • Primary prevention
- Cardiovascular disease

KEY POINTS

- There are millions of older adults with diabetes mellitus (DM) and there will be many more in the next 3 decades.
- Older adults with DM are at higher risk for morbidity and mortality related to atherosclerotic cardiovascular disease (ASCVD).
- Evidence-based clinical practice guidelines recommend lifestyle therapy plus moderate/high-intensity statin therapy to treat dyslipidemias to prevent ASCVD in people with DM 40 years to 75 years of age.
- A comprehensive approach is recommended to modify ASCVD risk factors that can be modified.
- Clinicians should discuss with patients greater than 75 years of age the risks and benefits of primary prevention of ASCVD.

INTRODUCTION

Globally, in 2017, there were an estimated 122.8 million (prevalence 9.6%) older adults (≥65 years of age) with diabetes mellitus (DM). By 2045, that number is projected to be 253.2 million (prevalence 17.9%).[1] In the United States, between 1997 and 2010, the number of older adults with DM rose from 4.20 million to 8.28 million.[2] In 2015, there were 12.0 million older adults with DM: 9.9 with diagnosed DM and 2.1 with

[a] Division of Metabolism, Endocrinology & Diabetes, Department of Internal Medicine, University of Michigan, 24 Frank Lloyd Wright Drive, Ann Arbor, MI 48105, USA; [b] Taubman Health Sciences Library, University of Michigan, 1135 Catherine Street, Ann Arbor, MI 48109, USA
* Corresponding author.
E-mail address: mengt@med.umich.edu

Clin Geriatr Med 36 (2020) 457–476
https://doi.org/10.1016/j.cger.2020.04.006   **geriatric.theclinics.com**
0749-0690/20/© 2020 Elsevier Inc. All rights reserved.

undiagnosed DM, representing approximately 40% of adults with DM.[3] Over the next 3 decades, that number is projected to increase significantly. Approximately 90% of older adults with DM have type 2 DM (T2DM). Many have had DM for more than a decade. The prevalence of coronary heart disease (CHD) and stroke is higher in them than in their counterparts without DM.[2] In a national survey of mortality in DM, 44% and 25% of death certificates listed ischemic heart disease and stroke, respectively, as cause of death.[4]

DM is a major risk factor for atherosclerotic cardiovascular disease (ASCVD)—CHD, stroke, and peripheral arterial disease.[5] Dyslipidemias and hypertension, other major risk factors, are common comorbidities in DM and further increase the risk for ASCVD in DM. Compared with their counterparts, people with DM with a myocardial infarction (MI) have a poorer prognosis and a higher CHD mortality rate either immediately or in the long term.[6,7]

Recent evidence-based clinical practice guidelines (CPGs) for the prevention of ASCVD in at-risk adults, with or without DM,[8–12] recommend a comprehensive approach to prevent ASCVD (**Fig. 1**). Evidence for CPG recommendations for people with DM come from subgroup analysis of data from subjects with DM in the cited randomized controlled trials (RCTs) except for 1 in which all subjects had DM. Furthermore, many subjects in these RCTs were adults without DM less than or equal to 75 years of age. Evidence for recommendations for older adults with DM is extrapolated from subgroup analysis of data from older subjects in these RCTs. This article focuses on the treatment of dyslipidemias in the primary prevention of ASCVD in older adults with DM.

DIABETES MELLITUS AND ATHEROSCLEROTIC CARDIOVASCULAR DISEASE CONNECTIONS

Box 1 summarizes selected connections between DM and ASCVD.[4,5,13–22]

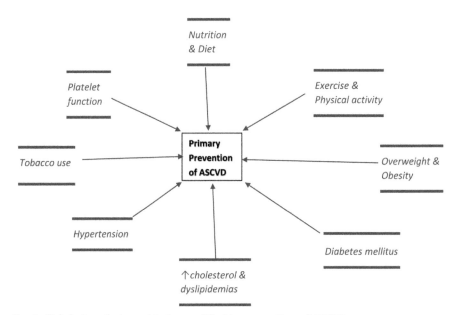

Fig. 1. Risk factors that need to be modified in prevention of ASCVD.

> **Box 1**
> **Summary of connections between diabetes mellitus and atherosclerotic cardiovascular disease**
>
> 1. People with DM are at higher risk for premature morbidity and mortality related to ASCVD.[5]
>
> 2. A meta-analysis of 102 prospective studies involving 698,782 patient records showed adjusted HRs, with 95% CIs, for ASCVD in people with DM were HR 2.00 (1.83–2.19) for CHD; HR 2.27 (1.95–2.65) for ischemic stroke; HR 1.56 (1.19–2.05) for hemorrhagic stroke; and HR 1.73 (1.51–1.98) deaths.[13]
>
> 3. In DM, women are affected by ASCVD more than men.[14]
>
> 4. People with DM have increased (×2–3) risk of mortality compared with people without DM,[16,17] and a majority of people (65%–80%) with DM die from ASCVD, specifically CHD and stroke.[4,15,18,19]
>
> 5. In the general older adult population, DM is a more common cause of death.[20]
>
> 6. Many deaths occur in people with DM with no prior signs or symptom of ASCVD. Furthermore, people with DM have a high prevalence of silent myocardial ischemia; and many had MIs without recognized or typical symptoms.[21]
>
> 7. People with DM have a shorter life expectancy partly because of premature ASCVD. In the United States, men and women with DM, age ≥50 years, have a shorter life expectancy by 7.5 years and 8.2 years, respectively, compared with their counterparts without DM.[22]

Primary Prevention of Atherosclerotic Cardiovascular Disease in Older Adults with Diabetes Mellitus

Primary prevention of ASCVD in older adults with DM is preventing the onset of their first event related to CHD (MI, acute coronary syndromes, angina, and coronary revascularization), cerebral arterial disease (stroke/transient ischemic attack), and peripheral arterial disease (claudication). Differentiating primary prevention and secondary prevention of ASCVD in people with DM can be challenging because they have a high prevalence of silent myocardial ischemia and MIs without recognized or typical symptoms.[18] There are ways to detect CHD in asymptomatic people with T2DM.[20] Although a recent meta-analysis of RCTs screening asymptomatic CHD in people with DM reported some benefits,[21] others do not recommend such screening.[22]

US CPGs recommend using risk calculators to estimate the risk level for developing ASCVD in the next 10 years as low (<5%), borderline (5%–7.5%), intermediate (≥7.5%–<20%), and high (≥20%) in individual patients and treat accordingly.[8,9]

Dyslipidemias—One of Many Major Risk Factors for Atherosclerotic Cardiovascular Disease in Diabetes Mellitus

People with T2DM have several major modifiable risk factors for ASCVD, including hyperglycemia, hypertension, and dyslipidemias. This article discusses only dyslipidemias and refers readers to the published CPGs[8–12] for evidence-based recommendations for other risk factors. **Box 2**[23–28] summarizes selected aspects of dyslipidemias in DM.

Efficacy and Safety of Statin Therapy for Dyslipidemias in the Prevention of Atherosclerotic Cardiovascular Disease

Table 1 summarizes selected meta-analyses of statin therapy to prevent ASCVD.[29–33] Statin therapy, efficacious and safe in primary prevention and secondary prevention, reduces major ASCVD events and mortality as well as all-cause mortality in patients

---

Box 2
Summary of features of dyslipidemias in diabetes mellitus

1. A majority of people with T2DM have dyslipidemia, which may or may not be present for years before the DM diagnosis.

2. The most common pattern for dyslipidemia is characterized by high TGs, reduced high-density lipoprotein cholesterol (HDL-C), and similar or slightly elevated LDL-C levels compared with those without DM.[23,24]

3. Their low-density lipoprotein (LDL) particles, besides being increased in concentration, are smaller, denser, and more susceptible to oxidation and glycation (because of the hyperglycemia), making them more atherogenic.

4. Their atherogenic index of plasma (AIP), a calculated plasma lipid index [log (TG/HDL-C)], is increased, as in people at higher risk for ASCVD, and inversely correlated with LDL particle size.[25] People with T2DM with high TGs, low HDL-C, and small LDL particle size also have increased AIP.[26]

5. In 2007 to 2010, in the United States, the mean (±SE) LDL-C in adults ≥65 years was 93.3 (2.52) mg/dL². In this group, 26.3 (2.71%) having an LDL-C <70; 36.9 (3.98%) LDL-C 70 to 99, 21.8 (3.00%) LDL-C 100 to 129; 10 (2.81%) LDL-C 130 to 159; and 5.1 (1.61%) LDL-C ≥160 mg/dL.

6. Although LDL-C usually is not greatly elevated in people with DM, it predicts CHD risk, as in the general population. In the UK Prospective Diabetes Study, a 1.57-fold increased risk of CHD was reported for every 1 mmol/L increment in LDL-C.[27] LDL-C also predicts stroke risk in people with T2DM.[28]

7. People with DM also may have familial dyslipidemias (hypercholesterolemia, combined dyslipidemia, or hypertriglyceridemia) as well as other secondary dyslipidemias (eg, hypothyroidism, end-stage renal disease, and others). In these people with combined diabetic and familial/other secondary dyslipidemias, the pattern of their dyslipidemia differs from the common pattern, described previously.

---

irrespective of their baseline low-density lipoprotein cholesterol (LDL-C) levels, sex, age and DM status. For every millimole/liter reduction of LDL-C, there is reduction of cardiovascular (CV) events by approximately 20%.

Efficacy of Statin Therapy in the Primary Prevention of Atherosclerotic Cardiovascular Disease in in People with Diabetes Mellitus

Table 2 shows selected RCTs on treating dyslipidemias with statin in primary prevention and secondary prevention of ASCVD in DM. The 4 RCTs that addressed primary prevention are discussed.

The Collaborative Atorvastatin Diabetes Study (CARDS) is the first primary prevention RCT in old people with T2DM without known CV disease (CVD) plus greater than or equal to 1 other ASCVD risk factor (retinopathy, albuminuria, current smoking, or hypertension).[34] Atorvastatin, 10 mg daily, reduced the risk of first CHD and stroke.

In the Heart Protection Study, primary prevention and secondary prevention of ASCVD were addressed in old people with DM.[35] In the 2912 DM subjects who had no known CHD at study entry, simvastatin, 40 mg daily, reduced the first major vascular event (MVE) by 33%. In the 2426 DM subjects with LDL-C less than 3.0 mmol/L (116 mg/dL), there was a reduction of 27%.

The Anglo-Scandinavian Cardiac Outcomes Trial—Lipid Lowering Arm (ASCOT-LLA) substudy enrolled 2532 old subjects with T2DM, hypertension, and greater than or equal to 3 risk factors.[36] In this DM subgroup, atorvastatin, 10 mg daily, reduced the incidence of total CV events.

Table 1
Summary of meta-analyses of clinical trials on the efficacy and safety of statin therapy to prevent atherosclerotic cardiovascular disease

Reference Median[a]/Mean[b] Follow-up Years	# CTs # Subjects	Findings (Rate Ratio 1.0 mmol/L LDL-C)	Safety
CTTC 2012 [29] 4.8[a] People with low CV risk	27 CTs N = 174,149 22 CTs (Sta vs Cont) N = 134,537 5 CTs (High vs Low) N = 39,612	MVE RR = 0.79(0.77–0.81; $P<.0001$) MCE: RR = 0.76(0.73–0.79; $P<.0001$) Stroke: RR = 0.85(0.80–0.89; $P<.0001$) CR: RR = 0.76(0.73–0.79; $P<.0001$) VM: RR = 0.85(0.77–0.95; $P = .004$) ACM: RR = 0.91(0.85–0.97; $P = .007$) PP MVE: RR = 0.75(0.70–0.80; $P<.0001$) SP MVE: RR = 0.80(0.77–0.82; $P<.0001$) Proportional ↓ MVE same in the 2 lowest and highest LDL-C categories.	Cancer incidence: RR = 1.0(0.96–1.04) Cancer mortality: RR = 0.99(0.93–1.06) N-VD: RR = 0.96 (0.92–1.01; $P = .16$)
CTTC 2015 [30] 4.8[a] Men vs Women	27 CTs N = 174,149 22 CTs (Sta vs Cont) N = 134,537 5 CTs (High vs Low) N = 39,612	Of 174,149 subjects, 27% were women. MVE: RR = 0.78(0.75–0.81)[c] Men RR = 0.84(0.74–0.91) Women PP MVE: RR = 0.72(0.66–0.80) Men RR = 0.85(0.72–1.00) Women SP MVE: RR = 0.79(0.76–0.82) Men RR = 0.84(0.77–0.91) Women Proportional ↓ % MVE similar <10% and >30% risk categories by 5 y vascular at baseline.	No significant effect on incident cancer or cancer mortality. No significant difference between men and women
CTTC 2010 [31] 4.8[a] More vs less statin intensity	26 CTs N = 169,138 21 CTs (Sta vs Cont) N = 129,526 5 CTs (High vs Low) N = 39,612	More vs less statin intensity trials (5 RCTs) More statin →0.51 mmol/L LDL-C ↓ vs less statin and further ↓MVE RR = 15% (11–18; $P<.0001$); ↓ NFMI or CD RR = 13% (7–1; $P<.0001$); ↓ CR RR = 19% (15–24; $P<.0001$); and ↓ Ischemic stroke RR = 16% (5–26; $P = 005$)	No significant ↑ in cancer incidence RR = 1.00(0.96–1.04; $P = .9$), cancer or other N-VD RR = 0.98 (0.81–1.18; $P = .8$)

(continued on next page)

Table 1
(continued)

Reference Median[a]/Mean[b] Follow-up Years	# CTs # Subjects	Findings (Rate Ratio 1.0 mmol/L LDL-C)	Safety
		All 26 trials results (by age groups) <65 y RR = 0.78(0.75–0.82) ≥65–75 y RR = 0.78(0.74–0.81) >75 y RR = 0.84(0.73–0.97)	
CTTC 2008 [32] 4.3[b] Diabetes mellitus	14 CTs DM = 18,686 (T1D = 1466 T2D = 17,220) NoDM = 71,370	MVE:DM RR = 0.79(0.72–0.86); NoDM: RR = 0.79(0.76–0.82) MCE: DM RR = 0.78(0.69–0.87); NoDM: RR = 0.77(0.73–0.81) CR: DM: RR = 0.75(0.64–0.88); NoDM: RR = 0.76(0.72–0.81) Stroke: DM: 0.79(0.67–0.93); NoDM: RR = 0.84(0.76–0.93) ACM:DM: 0.91(0.82–1.01; $P = .02$); NoDM: RR = 0.87(0.82–0.92; $P<.0001$) PP (DM): RR = 0.73(0.66–0.82); SP:(DM): RR = 0.80(0.74–0.88) PP(NoDM): RR = 0.78(0.71–0.81); SP(NoDM): RR = 0.79(0.76–0.82) MVE ≤65 y RR = 0.72(0.68–0.87); MVE >65 y RR = 0.81(0.71–0.92) After 5 y, 42 (30–55) fewer people with DM had MVE per 1000 allocated statin therapy. Reduction in MVE was 0.79(0.74–0.84) per mmol/L LDL-C reduction in DM total group and each baseline subgroups.	No information provided.
CTTC 2019 [33] 4.9[a] Older people	28 CTs N = 186,854 >75 y of age (N = 14,463)	MVE: >65-≤70y RR = 0.74(0.69–0.80); >70-≤75 y RR = 0.80(0.78–0.87); >75y RR = 0.82 (0.78–0.95)	No information provided.

(continued on next page)

Table 1 (continued)			
Reference **Median**[a]**/Mean**[b] **Follow-up Years**	**# CTs** **# Subjects**	**Findings (Rate Ratio** **1.0 mmol/L LDL-C)**	**Safety**
		MCE: >65-≤70y RR = 0.77(0.69–0.85); >70-≤75 y RR = 0.81(0.72–0.91); >75y RR = 0.82(0.70–0.96) CR: >65-≤70y RR = 0.69(0.62–0.77); >70-≤75y RR = 0.76(0.65–0.89); >75y RR = 1.02(0.75–1.40) STROKE: >65-≤70y RR = 0.83(0.72–0.96); >70-≤75y RR = 0.84 (0.72 0.96); >75y RR = 0.89(0.71–1.10) PP: >65-≤70y RR = 0.61(0.51–0.73); >70-≤75y RR = 0.84(0.70–1.01); >75y RR = 0.92(0.73–1.16) SP: >65-≤70y RR = 0.79(0.73–0.86); >70-≤75y RR = 0.80(0.73–0.88); >75y RR = 0.85(0.73–0.98)	

Abbreviations: #, number; ↑, increase; → results in; ↓, reduction; ACM, all-cause mortality; CD, coronary death; Cont, control; CR, coronary revascularization (%/annum); CTs, clinical trials; CTTC, Cholesterol Treatment Trialists' Collaboration; CV, cardiovascular; DM, diabetes mellitus; FU, follow-up; LDL-C, low density lipoprotein cholesterol; MCE, major coronary event (%/annum); MVE, major vascular event (%/annum); N, sample size; NFMI, non-fatal myocardial infarction; NoDM, no diabetes mellitus; N-VD, non-vascular deaths; PP, primary prevention; Ref, reference; RR, risk ratio (95% confidence interval); SP, secondary prevention; Sta, statin; Stroke, any stroke; T1D, type 1 diabetes; T2D, type 2 diabetes; VM, vascular mortality; y, year.

[a] Median.
[b] Mean.

The Atorvastatin Study for Prevention of Coronary Heart Disease Endpoints in Non-Insulin-Dependent Diabetes Mellitus (ASPEN)[37] addressed both primary prevention and secondary prevention of ASCVD in 2410 old T2DM subjects. Atorvastatin, 10 mg daily, did not reduce a composite clinical CV outcome endpoint.

In the Treating to New Targets study, a secondary prevention study, the atorvastatin, 80 mg daily, treatment subgroup of DM subjects lowered the LDL-C more and had fewer major CVD events compared with the atorvastatin, 10 mg daily, subgroup.[38] The greater the reduction of LDL-C, the greater the reduction in ASCVD events.

Finally, **Table 2** also includes 3 RCTs addressing only secondary prevention of ASCVD—4S substudy,[39] LIPID,[40] and CARE.[41] Readers are referred to the original articles for details.

Adding ezetimibe to simvastatin further lowered the LDL-C and resulted in greater reduction in the composite CV endpoint in IMPROVE-IT.[42] The benefit of

Table 2
Clinical trials on treating dyslipidemias to prevent atherosclerotic cardiovascular disease in diabetes mellitus

Study Name & Period, PP &/SP (Ref)	Intervention	Control	Sample Size Mean/Median Age Age(Range)	Follow-up Period	ASCVD End-Point	Relative Risk Reduction or Hazard Ratio (95% CI)	P-Value
Reduce LDL-C	*Statin only*						
CARDS 1997–2003, PP [34]	Atorvastatin 10 mg (N = 1428)	Placebo (N = 1410)	All T2DM 62 y (40–75) ~61–67% ≥60 y	~2 y Stopped 2 y early	MACE	MACE:0.63 = (0.48–0.83) CHD: 0.64 = (0.45–0.91) Stroke 0.52= (0.31–0.85)	P<.001 P<-.0001 P<.0001
HPS 1994–2001 PP & SP [35]	Simvastatin 40 mg (N = 10,269)	Placebo (N = 10,267)	DM: N = 5963 No DM: 14,573	5 y	Total CVD events	Total CVD events: 22% ([13–30])	P<.0001
ASCOT-LLA 1998–2003 PP [36]	Atorvastatin 10 mg (N = 1258)	Placebo (N = 1274)	T2DM: N = 2532 No DM N = 7773 ~64 y ~68%	3.9 y	Total CV Events & procedures (TCVE)	TCVE 0.77 (0.61–0.98)	P = .036
ASPEN 1996–2003 PP & SP [37]	Atorvastatin 10 mg (N = 1211)	Placebo (N = 1199)	All T2DM: N = 2420	4.25 y	Modified MACE	PP:0.97 (0.74–1.28) SP: 0.82(0.59–1.15)	NS NS
TNT (SP) 1998–2005 [38]	Atorvastatin 80 mg (N-748)	Atorvastatin 10 mg (N = 753)	T2DM: N = 1501 No DM: N = 8500 ~63 y (35–75)	4.9 y	Modified MACE	CV Events 0.85(0.75–0.97) Stroke 0.69(0.48–0.98) MACE 0.75(0.58–0.97)	P = .044 P = .037 P = .026
4S 1989–1994 SP [39]	Simvastatin 20–40 mg (n = 105)	Placebo (n = 97)	T2DM: N = 202 No DM: N = 4242 ~60 y (35–70)	5.4 y	Total mortality	CHD: 0.45(0.27–0.74)	P<.002
LIPID 1990–1997 SP 40	Pravastatin 40 mg (N = 396)	Placebo (N = 386)	DM: N = 782 No DM: N = 8232 62 (31–76)	6.1 y	CHD death	DM: 19(-11–41) No DM 25(15–33)	NS Significant
CARE 1989–1995 SP [41]	Pravastatin 40 mg (N = 282)	Placebo (N = 304)	DM: N = 586 No DM: N = 3573 ~60 y (21–75)	5 y	Fatal CHD/non-fatal MI	DM: 25(0–43) No DM:23(11–33)	P = .05 P<.001
Statin+ 1 other							

Trial	Treatment	Comparator	Population	Duration	Endpoint	Result	P value
IMPROVE-IT 2005–2012[42]	Simvatatin 40 mg + Ezetimibe (10 mg) (N = 2459)	Simvastatin 40 mg (N = 2474)	DM: N = 4933 No DM: N = 13,211 64 y (>50 y)	At least 2 y	Modified MACE	DM: 0.936(0.89–0.99)	P = .016
ODYSSEY (ODY) OUTCOMES Randomization 2012–2017 SP[43]	Alirocumab + statin (N = 2693)	Placebo + statin (N = 2751) 59 y	DM: (N = 5444) No DM (N = 5234) Pre DM (N = 8246)	Median 2.8 y	ODY MACE	DM 0.84(0.74–0.97) Ab RR 2.5 (0.4–4.2) No DM 0.85 (0.70–1.03) Ab RR 1,3(−0.3–3.7)	Significant Significant NS NS
FOURIER (F) DM Randomization 2013–2015 SP[44]	Evolocumab + statin (N = 5515)	Placebo + statin (N = 5516)	DM: (N = 11,031) No DM: (N = 165330)	Median of 2.2 y	F-PEP F-SEP	F-PEP: 0.83(0.75–0.93) F-SEC: 0.82(0.76–0.96)	P = 0008 P = .002
Lower TG							
Fibrate/IE							
FIELD 1998–2005 PP + SP[46]	Fenofibrate 200 mg (N-4895)	Placebo (N = 4900)	T2DM: N = 9795 62 y (50–75)	5 y	Non-fatal MI or CHD death	Coronary events 0.89 (0.75–1.05)	P = .16
ACCORD-Lipid 2001–2009[47]	Fenofibrate 160/54 mg + simvastatin (N = 2765)	Simvastatin 20–40 mg (N = 2753)	T2DM: N = 5518 ~62 y	4.7 y	Non-fatal MI/stroke/CHD death	MACE: 0.92 (0.79–1.08)	P = .32
REDUCE-IT 2011–2018 (PP & SP)[51]	Icosapient ethyl (IE) 4 gm daily + statin (N = 2394)	Placebo + Statin N = 2393	DM: N = 5878 No DM: N = 3389 64 y (57–69)	4.9 y	Modified MACE	DM: 0.77(0.68–0.87) No DM: 0.73(0.68–0.86)	Significant Significant

Abbreviations: 4S, Scandinavian Simvastatin Survival Study; Abs RR, absolute risk reduction; ACCORD-Lipid, Action to Control Cardiovascular Risk in Diabetes-Lipid; ASCOT-LLA, Anglo-Scandinavian Cardiac Outcomes Trial—Lipid Lowering Arm; ASCVD, atherosclerotic cardiovascular disease; ASPEN, Atorvastatin Study for Prevention of Coronary Heart Disease Endpoints in Non-Insulin-Dependent Diabetes Mellitus; CARDS, Collaborative Atorvastatin Diabetes Study; CARE, cholesterol and recurrent events; CHD, coronary heart disease; CVD, cardiovascular disease; DM, diabetes mellitus; FIELD, Fenofibrate Intervention and Event Lowering in Diabetes; HSP, Heart Protection Study; IMPROVE-IT, Improve Reduction of Outcomes: Vytorin Efficacy International Trial; LIPID, Long-term Intervention with Pravastatin in Ischaemic Disease; MACE, major adverse cardiac events; MI, myocardial infarction; NS, not significant; PEP, primary endpoint; PP, primary prevention; REDUCE-IT, Reduction of Cardiovascular Events with Icosapent Ethyl–Intervention; SEP, secondary endpoint; SP, secondary prevention; T2DM, Type 2 diabetes mellitus; TNT, treating to new targets; y, years.

simvastatin plus ezetimibe therapy appeared to be greater in DM subjects and in those greater than or equal to 75 years of age. Similarly, adding a proprotein convertase subtilisin/kexin type 9 (PCSK-9) inhibitor can lower LDL-C levels further and reduce ASCVD events.[43,44] These combination therapies usually are used in secondary prevention and, if indicated, also in primary prevention. Ezetimibe and PCSK-9 inhibitors can be used, instead of statin, for primary prevention in statin intolerant patients to lower their LDL-C.

When older patients with DM on statin therapy to reduce ASCVD risk have fasting triglycerides (TGs) greater than 500 mg/dL, they should be treated with fenofibrate and/or fish oil to reduce their risk of pancreatitis.[45] This risk for pancreatitis is not discussed further in this article. For ASCVD prevention in subjects with DM, fenofibrate treatment did not reduce the primary outcome in the Fenofibrate Intervention and Event Lowering in Diabetes (FIELD) study.[46] Similarly, in the ACCORD-Lipid study, adding fenofibrate to subjects with DM on statin therapy did not further reduce the endpoint of nonfatal MI, nonfatal stroke, or death from CV causes.[47]

Hypertriglyceridemia increases the risk for ASCVD.[48] After appropriate statin therapy for prevention of ASCVD, patients still have a significant residual ASCVD risk.[24] In them, hypertriglyceridemia indicates an increased risk for ischemic CV event in elderly subjects (median age, 66 years)[49] and elderly subjects (mean age, 64 years) with DM.[50] In the Reduction of Cardiovascular Events with Icosapent Ethyl–Intervention Trial (REDUCE-IT), a majority of the subjects had DM and were elderly. Adding icosapent ethyl to statin to lower elevated serum TGs (135–499 mg/dL) significantly reduced the primary efficacy composite endpoint in subjects with DM.[51] Recently, an advisory panel recommended adding n-3 fatty acids (eicosapentaenoic acid [EPA] + docosahexaenoic acid [DHA] or EPA-only) at a dose of 4 g/d (>3 g/d total EPA + DHA) as an efficacious and safe option for reducing TGs as monotherapy or as an adjunct to other lipid-lowering medications, as this was not in the 2019 CPGs.[52] Lowering elevated TGs with n-3 fatty acids (EPA + DHA 4 g/d in older adults with DM on appropriate statin therapy) is another therapeutic step to consider.

Efficacy and Safety of Statin Therapy in Older and Very Old Adults

Table 3 summarizes 3 RCTs[53–56] and meta-analyses of 3 RCTs[33,57,58] in older and very old (>75 years of age) adults with or without DM using statins to prevent ASCVD. Overall, the data suggest that statins are efficacious and safe in both primary prevention and secondary prevention of ASCVD in the 65-year-old to 75-year-old group. In the greater than 75-year-old group, the reduction in MVEs in primary prevention for the total group and for any stroke are not statistically significant in the meta-analysis.[33]

Currently, there are limited data available on statin therapy for primary prevention of ASCVD in the very old adults. Statins for Reducing Events in the Elderly (STAREE)[59] is a primary prevention trial recruiting 18,000 subjects greater than 70 years of age to determine the efficacy, safety, and quality of life benefits of atorvastatin, 40 mg daily. Its primary endpoint is either the time from randomization to (1) death or development of dementia or (2) a major fatal or nonfatal CV event. When completed, it hopefully will uncover new information on the efficacy and safety of statin in this very old group.

Recently a large observational study involving 46,864 participants (mean age 77 years) reported that participants with DM and on statin had a hazard ratio (HR) 0.76 (0.65–0.94) for ASCVD and HR 0.84 (0.75–0.94) for all-cause mortality in the 75-year-old to 84-year-old group.[60] In those ages greater than or equal to 85 years old, HRs were 0.82 (0.53–1.26) for ASCVD and 1.95(0.86–1.28) for all-cause mortality.

As for safety, the RCTs show that long-term statin therapy can lead to serious adverse events, such as myopathy, incident DM, and, probably, hemorrhagic

Table 3
Randomized control trials and meta-analysis of clinical trials using statin in the prevention of ASCVD in older adults

Reference (Year)	Sample Size Mean/Median Age (Years)	Years of Follow-up Median/Mean	Type of Prevention	Safety Findings	Endpoints: Hazard Ratio; Relative Risk, or Risk Ratio, all with (95% Confidence Intervals)
	Randomized controlled trials				
Shephard et al (2002) PROSPER [53], Llyod et al (2013)	N = 5804 70–82 y with mean age = 75.4 y	Mean 3.2 y	Primary Secondary	Incident cancer ↑ during trial (53). Follow-up of 8.6 y showed no ↑ in cancer (P = .22). (54)	Composite of coronary death, non-fatal MI, and fatal/non-fatal stroke. HR = 0.85 (0.74–0.97; P = .014). CHD death & non-fatal MI risk was reduced HR = 0·81 (0·69–0·94, P = .006). Stroke risk was not: HR = 1·03 (0·81–1·31; P = .8)
Ridker P et al (2008) JUPITER [55]	N-17802 Median age = 66 y	Median 1.9 y	Primary	No difference in incident cancer, muscle, GI, Hepatic & renal function. ↑ in incident DM.	Composite of nonfatal MI/stroke, CV death, hospitalization for unstable angina or revascularization: HR = 0.56 (0.46–0.69; P<.00001)

(continued on next page)

Table 3
(continued)

Reference (Year)	Sample Size Mean/Median Age (Years)	Years of Follow-up Median/Mean	Type of Prevention	Safety Findings	Endpoints: Hazard Ratio; Relative Risk, or Risk Ratio, all with (95% Confidence Intervals)
Yusof S et al (2016) HOPE-3 [56]	N = 12,705 Mean age = 66 y	Median 5.0 y	Primary	Rosuvastatin 10 mg: ↓ admissions for CV causes & deep vein thrombosis. More cataract surgery & muscle complaints.	Total group 1st composite end point of CV death, nonfatal MI, or nonfatal stroke: HR = 0.76 (0.64–0.91; P = .002) 2nd composite end point of 1st end point + resuscitated cardiac arrest, heart failure, or revascularization. HR = 0.75 (0.64–0.91; P<.001)
Meta-analysis					
Savanese et al (2013) [57]	8 CTs, N = 24,674 Mean age = 73 y	Mean 5.5 y	Primary	Cancer 0.99 (0.85–1.15)	MI Rel R = 0.61(0.43–0.85) Stroke Rel R = 0.76 (0.63–0.93) CV death Rel R = 0.91 (0.69–1.20)
Ridker P et al (2017) [58]	2 CTs, (JUPITER & HOPE 3), >70 y groups JUPITER N = 5695 HOPE-3 N = 3086		Primary		Composite of nonfatal MI, nonfatal stroke or CV death HR = 0.74 (0.61–0.91)

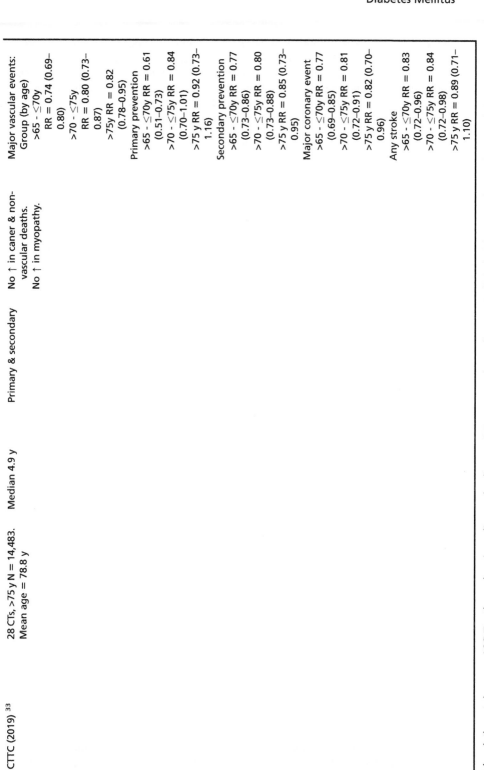

CTTC (2019) [33]	28 CTs, >75 y N = 14,483. Mean age = 78.8 y	Median 4.9 y	Primary & secondary	No ↑ in caner & non-vascular deaths. No ↑ in myopathy.	Major vascular events: Group (by age) >65 - ≤70y RR = 0.74 (0.69–0.80) >70 - ≤75y RR = 0.80 (0.73–0.87) >75y RR = 0.82 (0.78–0.95) Primary prevention >65 - ≤70y RR = 0.61 (0.51–0.73) >70 - ≤75y RR = 0.84 (0.70–1.01) >75 y RR = 0.92 (0.73–1.16) Secondary prevention >65 - ≤70y RR = 0.77 (0.73–0.86) >70 - ≤75y RR = 0.80 (0.73–0.88) >75 y RR = 0.85 (0.73–0.95) Major coronary event >65 - ≤70y RR = 0.77 (0.69–0.85) >70 - ≤75y RR = 0.81 (0.72–0.91) >75 y RR = 0.82 (0.70–0.96) Any stroke >65 - ≤70y RR = 0.83 (0.72–0.96) >70 - ≤75y RR = 0.84 (0.72–0.98) >75 y RR = 0.89 (0.71–1.10)

Abbreviations: ↑, increase; ASCVD, atherosclerotic cardiovascular disease; CHD, coronary heart disease; CT, clinical trials; CV, cardiovascular; DM, diabetes mellitus; GI, gastrointestinal; HOPE-3, heart outcomes prevention evaluation; HR, hazard ratio (95% confidence intervals); JUPITER, Justification for the Use of Statins in Prevention: an Intervention Trial Evaluating Rosuvastatin; MI, myocardial infarction; CTs, randomized controlled trials; Rel R, relative risk; RR, risk ratio; y, years.

stroke.[61] The RCTs conducted in older adults in **Table 3** did not report any concerning adverse events except in the PROspective Study of Pravastatin in the Elderly at Risk. (PROSPER) study, which reported an increase in incident cancer during the study period.[53] During 8.6 years of follow-up, however, there was no increase in incident cancer.[54] In older adults a decline in cognitive function would be concerning, but statins have not been definitively linked with cognitive impairment.[62]

Clinical Practice Guidelines for Treating Dyslipidemias in the Primary Prevention of Atherosclerotic Cardiovascular Disease

Relevant CPGs on treating dyslipidemias to prevent ASCVD in adults, with and without DM, have been published in the United States.[8-11] Of these, only 1 specifically addressed treating dyslipidemias in older adults with DM.[11] For successful prevention of ASCVD, a comprehensive approach in modifying risk factors that can be modified (see **Fig. 1**) is recommended.[63]

All 5 CPGs published in 2019 recommended basically the same approach, with variations, for prevention of ASCVD.[8-12] When treating dyslipidemia in the primary prevention of ASCVD in older adults with DM, the clinician first assesses a patient's major ASCVD risk factors profile and ASCVD risk enhancers.[8,9] Secondly, the 10-year risk for ASCVD using a risk factor calculator[8-11] is estimated and categorized as low, borderline, intermediate, and high. One CPG categorize the risk groups without a risk calculator.[12] All CPGs advocate lifestyle therapy (diet and physical activity) plus pharmacotherapy. Almost all older adults with DM have intermediate risk or high risk for ASCVD (**Fig. 2**). The prescribed statin (moderate intensity or high intensity [**Table 4**]) is dependent on whether a patient is at intermediate risk or high risk for developing ASCVD in the next 10 years.

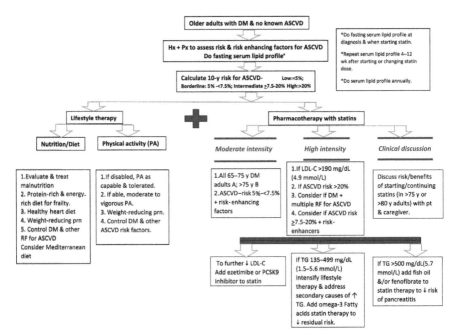

Fig. 2. An approach to treating dyslipidemias in older adults with DM for primary prevention of ASCVD. A, 65-75y DM adults; B, >75y; Hx, history; Px, physical examination; PA, physical activity; Pt, patient; prn, as needed; RF, risk factors.

| | **Table 4** | | |
| | **Statins dosing according to intensity of therapy** | | |
Generic Name	**Low-Intensity Treatment (Daily Dose Decreases Low-Density Lipoprotein Cholesterol by <30% on Average)**	**Moderate-Intensity Treatment (Daily Dose Decreases Low-Density Lipoprotein Cholesterol by 30%–50% on Average)**	**High-Intensity Treatment (Daily Dose Decreases Low-Density Lipoprotein Cholesterol by >50% on Average)**
Atorvastatin	10 mg	10–40 mg	40–80 mg
Fluvastatin	20–40 mg	80 mg	—
Lovastatin	10–20 mg	40–80 mg	—
Pitastatin	1 mg	2–4 mg	—
Pravastatin[a]	10–20 mg	40–80 mg	—
Rouvastatin	5 mg	5–10 mg	10–40 mg
Simvastatin[a]	5–10 mg	20–40 mg	—

[a] To be taken at bedtime.

CPGs recommend a discussion between clinician and patient regarding risks/benefits of statin therapy for the very old (>75 years of age). When such a person has been taking statin for years before and has experienced no adverse events, should the statin be deprescribed because of chronologic age? A recent study reported statin discontinuation was associated with a 33% increased risk of admission for CV event in these primary prevention patients.[64] Ongoing statin therapy can be continued in these greater than 75 year old patients if they are otherwise healthy[65]

SUMMARY

Older adults with DM are at higher risk for morbidity and mortality related to ASCVD. Based on evidence for the efficacy and safety of statins to prevent ASCVD in adults, CPGs[8–12] recommend statin therapy for people with DM from age 40 years to 75 years using either moderate-intensity or high-intensity statin doses, depending on risk. The evidence for those greater than 75 years of age, with or without DM, is limited at present. No stand-alone RCT, like CARDS, for primary prevention of ASCVD, in this age group has been completed.

Older adults with DM, like those without DM of comparable age, may have other health and social problems (comorbidities, shorter life span, physical disability, cognitive impairment, sarcopenia, frailty, polypharmacy, and more), which should be considered when deciding ASCVD primary prevention plans.[65,66] Each plan should be discussed with the older adults with DM and their caregivers. Uncertainties about the benefits and harms of statins for primary ASCVD prevention in adults ages greater than 75 years, especially those with other health and/or social issues, remain until new knowledge from RCTs is uncovered.[67,68] If implemented, a comprehensive approach, not just targeting dyslipidemia, should be used in otherwise healthy greater than 75 years of age adults with DM.

DISCLOSURE

The authors have nothing to disclose.

REFERENCES

1. IDF diabetes Atlas – International diabetes Federation. Available at: https://diabetesatlas.org/resources/2017-atlas.htm. Accessed October 15, 2019.

2. Laiteerapong N, Huang ES. Chapter 16: diabetes in older adults. In: Cowie CC, Casagrande SS, Menke A, et al, editors. Diabetes in America. 3rd edition. Bethesda (MD): National Institutes of Health, NIH Pub No. 17-1468; 2017. p. 16–26.

3. Centers for Disease Control and Prevention. National diabetes statistics report, 2017. Atlanta (GA): Centers for Disease Control and Prevention, U.S. Dept of Health and Human Services; 2017.

4. Gu K, Cowie CC, Harris MI. Mortality in adults with and without diabetes in a national cohort of the U.S. Population,1971-1993. Diabetes Care 1998;21:1138–45.

5. Almdal T, Scharling H, Jensen JS, et al. The independent effect of type 2 diabetes mellitus on ischemic heart disease, stroke, and death: a population-based study of 13,000 men and women with 20 years of follow-up. Arch Intern Med 2004;164: 1422–6.

6. Haffner SM, Lehto S, Ronnemaa T, et al. Mortality from coronary heart disease in subjects with type 2 diabetes and in nondiabetic subjects with and without prior myocardial infarction. N Engl J Med 1998;339:229–34.

7. Miettinen H, Lehto S, Salomaa V, et al. Impact of diabetes on mortality after the first myocardial infarction: the FINMONICA myocardial infarction Register study group. Diabetes Care 1998;21:69–75.

8. Grundy SM, Stone NJ, Bailey AL, et al. AHA/ACC/AACVPR/AAPA/ABC/ACPM/ADA/AGS/APhA/ASPC/NLA/PCNA guideline on the management of blood cholesterol: a report of the American College of Cardiology/American heart association Task Force on clinical practice guidelines. J Am Coll Cardiol 2019;73: 285–350.

9. Arnett DK, Blumenthal RS, Albert MA, et al. 2019 ACC/AHA guideline on the primary prevention of cardiovascular disease A report of the American College of Cardiology/American heart association Task Force on clinical practice guidelines. J Am Coll Cardiol 2019;74:e177–232.

10. American Diabetes Association. Cardiovascular disease and risk management: classification and diagnosis of diabetes: standards of medical care in diabetes-2019. Diabetes Care 2019;42(Suppl 1):S103–23.

11. LeRoith D, Biessels GJ, Braidwaithe SS, et al. Treatment of diabetes in older adults: an endocrine society clinical practice guideline. J Clin Endocrinol Metab 2019;104:1520–74.

12. Consentino F, Grant PJ, Aboyans V, et al. 2019 ESC Guidelines on diabetes, prediabetes, and cardiovascular diseases developed in collaboration with the EASD. Eur Heart J 2020;41(2):255–323.

13. Sarwar N, Gao P, Seshasai SR, et al. Emerging Risk Factors Collaboration: diabetes mellitus, fasting blood glucose concentration, and risk of vascular disease: a collaborative meta-analysis of 102 prospective studies. Lancet 2010;375: 2215–22.

14. Lee WL, Cheung AM, Cape D, et al. Impact of diabetes on coronary artery disease in women and men: a meta-analysis of prospective studies. Diabetes Care 2000;23:962–8.

15. Taylor KS, Heneghan CJ, Farmer AJ, et al. All-cause and cardiovascular mortality in middle-aged people with type 2 diabetes compared with people without diabetes in a large U.K. primary care database. Diabetes Care 2013;36:2366–71.

16. Li S, Wang J, Zhang B, et al. Diabetes mellitus and cause-specific mortality: a population-based study. Diabetes Metab J 2019;43:319–41.
17. Rosenquist KJ, Fox CS. Mortality trends in type 2 diabetes. In: Cowie CC, Casagrande SS, Menke A, et al, editors. Ch 36 in diabetes in America. 3rd edition. Bethesda (MD): National Institutes of Health; 2018. p. 1–14.
18. Cohn PF, Fox KM, Daly C. Silent myocardial ischemia. Circulation 2003;108: 1263–77.
19. Franco OH, Steyerberg EW, Hu FB, et al. Associations of diabetes mellitus with total life expectancy and life expectancy with and without cardiovascular disease. Arch Intern Med 2007;167:1145–51.
20. Djaberi R, Beishuizen ED, Pereira AM, et al. Non-invasive cardiac imaging techniques and vascular tools for the assessment of cardiovascular disease in type 2 diabetes mellitus. Diabetologia 2008;51:1581–93.
21. Clerc OF, Fuchs TA, Stehli J, et al. Non-invasive screening for coronary artery disease in asymptomatic diabetic patients: a systematic review and meta-analysis of randomized controlled trials. Eur Heart J Cardiovasc Imaging 2018;19:838–46.
22. Rados DV, Pinto LC, Leitão CB, et al. Screening for coronary artery disease in patients with type 2 diabetes: a meta-analysis and trial sequential analysis. BMJ Open 2017;7(5):e015089.
23. Rana JS, Liu JY, Moffet HH, et al. Metabolic dyslipidemia and risk of coronary heart disease in 28,318 adults with diabetes mellitus and low-density lipoprotein cholesterol <100 mg/dl. Am J Cardiol 2015;116:1700–4.
24. Fruchart JC, Sacks FM, Hermans MP, et al. The Residual Risk Reduction Initiative: a call to action to reduce residual vascular risk in dyslipidaemic patient. Diab Vasc Dis Res 2008;5:319–35.
25. Dobiasova M, Frohlich J. The plasma parameter log (TG/HDL-C) as an atherogenic index: correlation with lipoprotein particle size and esterification rate in apo B-lipoprotein-depleted plasma (FERHDL). Clin Biochem 2001;34:583–8.
26. Tan MH, Johns D, Glazer NB. Pioglitazone reduces atherogenic index of plasma in patients with type 2 diabetes. Clin Chem 2004;50:1184–8.
27. Turner RC, Millns H, Neil HA, et al. Risk factors for coronary artery disease in non-insulin dependent diabetes mellitus: United Kingdom Prospective Diabetes Study (UKPDS: 23). BMJ 1998;316:823–8.
28. Kothari V, Stevens RJ, Adler AI, et al. Ukpds 60: risk of stroke in type 2 diabetes estimated by the UK Prospective Diabetes Study risk engine. Stroke 2002;33: 1776–81.
29. Cholesterol Treatment Trialists' (CTT) Collaborators. The effects of lowering LDL cholesterol with statin therapy in people at low risk of vascular disease: meta-analysis of individual data from 27 randomised trials. Lancet 2012;380:581–90.
30. Cholesterol Treatment Trialists' (CTT) Collaborators. Efficacy and safety of LDL-lowering therapy among men and women: meta-analysis of individual data from174 000 participants in 27 randomised trials. Lancet 2015;385:1397–405.
31. Cholesterol Treatment Trialists' (CTT) Collaborators. Efficacy and safety of more intensive lowering of LDL cholesterol: a meta-analysis of data from 170 000 participants in 26 randomised trials. Lancet 2015;376:1670–81.
32. Cholesterol Treatment Trialists' Collaborators. Efficacy of cholesterol-lowering therapy in 18 686 people with diabetes in 14 randomised trials of statins: a meta-analysis. Lancet 2008;371:117–25.
33. Cholesterol Treatment Trialists' (CTT) Collaborators. Efficacy and safety of statin therapy in older people: a meta-analysis of individual participant data from 28 randomised controlled trials. Lancet 2019;393:407–15.

34. Colhoun HM, Betteridge DJ, Durrington PN, et al. Primary prevention of cardio-vascular disease with atorvastatin in type 2 diabetes in the Collaborative Atorvastatin Diabetes Study (CARDS): multicentre randomised placebo-controlled trial. Lancet 2004;364:685–696.35.

35. Collins R, Armitage J, Parish S, et al, Heart Protection Study Collaborative Group. MRC/BHF Heart Protection Study of cholesterol-lowering with simvastatin in 5963 people with diabetes: a randomised placebo-controlled trial. Lancet 2003;361: 2005–16.

36. Sever PS, Poulter NR, Dahl B, et al. Reduction in cardiovascular events with ator-vastatin in 2,532 patients with type 2 diabetes: anglo-scandinavian cardiac out-comes trial–lipid-lowering arm (ASCOT-LLA. Diabetes Care 2005;28:18–151–157.

37. Knopp RH, d'Emden M, Smilde JG, et al. Efficacy and safety of atorvastatin in the prevention of cardiovascular end points in subjects with type 2 diabetes: the Ator-vastatin Study for Prevention of Coronary Heart Disease Endpoints in non-insulin-dependent diabetes mellitus (ASPEN). Diabetes Care 2006;29:1478–838.

38. Shepherd J, Barter P, Carmena R, et al. Effect of lowering LDL cholesterol sub-stantially below currently recommended levels in patients with coronary heart dis-ease and diabetes: the Treating to New Targets (TNT) study. Diabetes Care 2006; 29:1220–6.

39. Pyörala K, Pedersen TR, Kjekshus J, et al. Cholesterol lowering with simvastatin improves prognosis of diabetic patients with coronary heart disease. A subgroup analysis of the Scandinavian Simvastatin Survival Study (4S). Diabetes Care 1997;20:614–20.

40. Long-Term Intervention with Pravastatin in Ischaemic Disease (LIPID) Study Group. Prevention of cardiovascular events and death with pravastatin in patients with coronary heart disease and a broad range of initial cholesterol levels. N Engl J Med 1998;339:1349–57.

41. Goldberg RB, Mellies MJ, Sacks FM, et al, The CARE Investigators. Cardiovascu-lar events and their reduction with pravastatin in diabetic and glucose-intolerant myocardial infarction survivors with average cholesterol levels: subgroup ana-lyses in the Cholesterol and Recurrent Events (CARE) trial. Circulation 1998; 98(23):2513–9.

42. Cannon CP, Braunwald E, McCabe CH, et al. Intensive versus moderate lipid lowering with statins after acute coronary syndromes. N Engl J Med 2004;350: 1495–504.

43. Sabatine MC, Leiter LA, Wiviott SD, et al. Cardiovascular safety and efficacy of the PCSK9 inhibitor evolocumab in patients with and without diabetes and the ef-fect of evolocumab on glycaemia and risk of new-onset diabetes: a prespecified analysis of the FOURIER randomized controlled trial. Lancet Diabetes Endocrinol 2017;5:941–50.

44. Ray KK, Colhoun HM, Szarek M, et al. Effects of alirocumab on cardiovascular and metabolic outcomes after acute coronary syndrome in patients with or without diabetes: a prespecified analysis of the ODYSSEY OUTCOMES rando-mised controlled trial. Lancet Diabetes Endocrinol 2019;7:618–28.

45. Chaudhary A, Iqbal U, Anwar H, et al. Acute pancreatitis secondary to severe hy-pertriglyceridemia: management of severe hypertriglyceridemia in emergency setting. Gastroenterol Res 2017;10(3):190–2.

46. The FIELD study investigators. Effects of long-term fenofibrate therapy on cardio-vascular events in 9795 people with type 2 diabetes mellitus (the FIELD study): randomised controlled trial. Lancet 2005;366:1849–61.

47. The ACCORD Study Group. Effects of combination lipid therapy in type 2 diabetes mellitus. N Engl J Med 2010;362:1563–74.
48. Nordestgaard BG. Triglyceride-rich lipoproteins and atherosclerotic cardiovascular disease new insights from epidemiology, genetics, and biology. Circ Res 2016;118:547–63.
49. Nichols GA, Philip S, Reynolds K, et al. Increased cardiovascular risk in hypertriglyceridemic patients with statin-controlled LDL cholesterol. J Clin Endocrinol Metab 2018;103:3019–27.
50. Nichols GA, Philip S, Reynolds K, et al. Increased residual cardiovascular risk in patients with diabetes and high versus normal triglycerides despite statin-controlled LDL cholesterol. Diabetes Obes Metab 2018;21:366–71.
51. Bhatt DL, Steg PG, Miller M, et al. Cardiovascular risk reduction with icosapent ethyl for hypertriglyceridemia. N Engl J Med 2019;380:11–22.
52. Skulas-Ray AC, Wilson PWF, Harris WS, et al. Omega-3 fatty acids for the management of hypertriglyceridemia. a science advisory from the American Heart Association. Circulation 2019;140:e673–91.
53. Shephard J, Blauw GJ, Murphy MB, et al. Pravastatin in elderly individuals at risk of vascular disease (PROSPER): a randomised controlled trial. Lancet 2002;360:1623–30.
54. Lloyd SM, Stott DJ, de Craen AJ, et al. Long-term effects of statin treatment in elderly people: extended follow-up of the Prospective Study of Pravastatin in the Elderly at Risk (PROSPER). PLoS One 2013;8:e72642.
55. Ridker PM, Danielson E, Francisco AH, et al. Rosuvastatin to prevent vascular events in men and women with elevated C-reactive protein. N Engl J Med 2008;359:2195–207.
56. Yusof S, Bosch J, Dagenais G, et al. Cholesterol lowering in intermediate-risk persons without cardiovascular disease. N Engl J Med 2016;374:2021–31.
57. Savarese G, Gotto AM Jr, Paolillo S, et al. Benefits of statins in elderly subjects without established cardiovascular disease. A meta-analysis. J Am Coll Cardiol 2013;62:2090–9.
58. Ridker PM, Lonn E, Paynter NP, et al. Primary prevention with statin theray in the elderly. new meta-analyses from the contemporary JUPITER and HOPE-3 randomized trials. Circulation 2017;135:1979–81.
59. Available at: https://clinicaltrials.gov/ct2/show/NCT02099123. Accessed October 15, 2019.
60. Ramos R, Comas-Cuff M, Marti-Llich R, et al. Statins for primary prevention of cardiovascular events and mortality in old and very old adults with and without type 2 diabetes: retrospective cohort study. BMJ 2018;362:k3359.
61. Collins R, Reith C, Emberson J, et al. Interpretation of the evidence for the efficacy and safety of statin therapy. Lancet 2016;388:2532–61.
62. Adhyaru BB, Jacobson TA. Safety and efficacy of statin therapy. Nat Rev Cardiol 2018;15:757–61.
63. Gaede P, Lund-Andersen H, Parving HH, et al. Effect of a multifactorial intervention on mortality in type 2 diabetes. N Engl J Med 2008;358:580–91.
64. Giral P, Neumann A, Weill A, et al. Cardiovascular effect of discontinuing statins for primary prevention at the age of 75 years: a nationwide population-based cohort study in France. Eur Heart J 2019;40(43):3516–25.
65. Strandberg TM. Role of statin therapy in primary prevention of cardiovascular disease in elderly patients. Curr Atheroscler Rep 2019;21:28.
66. Mortensen MB, Falk E. Primary prevention with statins in the elderly. J Am Coll Cardiol 2018;71:85–94.

67. Singh S, Zieman S, Go AS, et al. Statins for primary prevention in older adults. Moving toward evidence-based decision-making. J Am Geriatr Soc 2018;66: 2188–96.
68. Hawley CE, Roefaro J, Forman DE, et al. Statins for primary prevention in those aged 70 years and older: a critical review of recent cholesterol guidelines. Drugs Aging 2019;26:687–99.

Improving Adherence in Type 2 Diabetes

Khine Swe, MD[a,b], S. Sethu K. Reddy, MD, MBA[b,*]

KEYWORDS

- Primary nonadherence • Secondary nonadherence • Medication persistence
- Shared decision making

KEY POINTS

- Primary nonadherence occurs when a patient never fills a prescription or never initially begins a medication.
- Secondary nonadherence occurs when a patient starts a medication for some time but later becomes nonadherent.
- Nonadherence with diabetes may be affected by treatment characteristics and complexity, age, gender, self-esteem, stress, depression, and quality of the patient-clinician relationship.
- Nonadherence, along with suboptimal prescribing, drug administration, and diagnosis, costs the health care system as much as $290 billion per year—or 13% of total health care expenditures.
- Personalized multifaceted intervention strategies, including technology solutions, are necessary to impact medication adherence.

INTRODUCTION

Although clinical trials show benefits of therapies, their effectiveness is more limited in real-life clinical settings. Clinicians tend to overestimate adherence rates among their own patients. Heightened awareness of nonadherence and new methodologies to improve adherence will usher in a new age of personalized diabetes care.

Type 2 diabetes mellitus (T2DM) is a highly prevalent, chronic metabolic disease with tremendous public health and socioeconomic implications. The recent report by the International Diabetes Federation estimates suggest that there are more than a half-billion adults ages 20 years to 79 years worldwide who have diabetes mellitus (DM) and that the global health care expenditure for adults with DM in 2015 was $673 billion.

There is strong evidence that improved glycemic control (lowering hemoglobin A_{1c} to $\leq 7\%$) can reduce the risk of microvascular and macrovascular complications. It also is known that many patients with diabetes are not achieving optimal glucose

[a] St. Mary's Ascension, CMU College of Medicine, Saginaw, MI, USA; [b] Department of Internal Medicine, CMED 2419, Central Michigan University, Mt. Pleasant, MI 48859, USA
* Corresponding author.
E-mail address: reddy3s@cmich.edu

Clin Geriatr Med 36 (2020) 477–489
https://doi.org/10.1016/j.cger.2020.04.007
0749-0690/20/© 2020 Elsevier Inc. All rights reserved.

geriatric.theclinics.com

control and many more are not reaching their targets for blood pressure and cholesterol. From numerous studies, it seems that fewer than 20% of those with diabetes attain hemoglobin A_{1c}, blood pressure, and cholesterol targets together. Improved glycemic control also may have a beneficial economic impact. Using the CORE Diabetes Model in the United Kingdom, modest improvements in glycemic control for 5 years led to a cost avoidance of £340 million.[1] An important barrier to achieving optimal metabolic control is nonadherence to recommended lifestyle changes and/ or prescribed medication regimens.

Many factors affect adherence to treatment in diabetes, such as disease and treatment characteristics and complexity, age, gender, self-esteem, stress, depression, quality of the relationship between patients and health care providers, social support, and patients' ability to remain adherent in the middle of daily stresses.

Compounding the issue of nonadherence is age range changes in demographics. The world is facing an aging phenomenon; in 2015, 901 million people were aged greater than or equal to 60 years, with most of these individuals living in developed countries. This number is expected to more than double by 2050, reaching 2.1 billion (ie, 20% of the global population). Moreover, the number of people aged greater than 80 years is growing more rapidly than the general elderly population. Approximately 14% of the elderly population (125 million) were greater than or equal to 80 years in 2015, and this number is expected to triple by 2050, reaching 434 million (approximately 20% of the senior population)[1,2] This phenomenon puts clear pressure on health care systems and social service support structures. Older adults typically exhibit the co-occurrence of multiple conditions and chronic diseases (including diabetes), which makes their care, in particular their use of medications, a challenging task. More than 90% of older adults are prescribed drugs, 50% of whom take 5 or more drugs and 10% of whom take 10 or more.[3] Prevalence of polypharmacy (defined as at least 5 prescribed medications) in the elderly increases with age. It is reported that 36% to 49% of patients greater than 75 years are prescribed polymedication, with differences related to the cohort considered and to nationality.[4] Nonadherence to medication and to medical plans, in general, are well-recognized public health problems. It is a challenge for researchers and health care providers because numerous efforts to improve patient adherence and persistence seem ineffective.[5] This is important particularly in older adults due to the high number of coexisting chronic diseases and geriatric syndromes.

DEFINITION OF ADHERENCE

Patients do not always take their medication as advised. Forgetfully or deliberately, they miss doses or do not follow the instructions. Occasionally, they stop taking a prescribed medication altogether.[6] These behaviors have huge ramifications on both health care quality and cost.[7] In 2003, the World Health Organization (WHO) identified medication nonadherence as the leading cause of preventable morbidity, mortality, and health care costs.[8] The WHO reviewed the literature on secondary nonadherence to chronic disease prescription medications and concluded the following: (1) medications do not work if patients do not take them, (2) medication nonadherence is a worldwide problem that crosses all jurisdictions, (3) the prevalence of medication nonadherence is of striking magnitude, and (4) this complex issue should be an urgent priority for policy makers and health care providers.[9]

Two important patient behaviors to help achieve good glycemic control include adherence (the extent to which a medication is taken at the prescribed doses, intervals, and frequency) and persistence (continuation of treatment for the prescribed duration).[10]

Medication adherence refers to the act of conforming to the recommendations made by the provider with respect to timing, dosage, and frequency of medication taking. Therefore, medication compliance may be defined as "the extent to which a patient acts in accordance with the prescribed interval and dose of a dosing regimen."[10] Persistence is operationalized in retrospective assessments as the number of doses dispensed in relation to the dispensing period, often called the medication possession ratio (MPR).[11] Persistence is reported as a continuous variable in terms of number of days for which therapy was available. Persistence also may be reported as a dichotomous variable measured at the end of a predefined time period (eg, 12 months), considering patients as being persistent or nonpersistent. MPR generally is calculated as the number of days for which the medication is supplied divided by the number of days in the study period. Calculation of proportion of days covered (PDC) is by dividing the number of days medication available to the patient by the number of days in the follow-up period multiplied by 100 and capped at 1. Adherence was defined in most studies as an MPR or PDC of greater than or equal to 0.80. For example, if a patient only filled one 3-month supply of medication over a 6-month period, then the patient is deemed as having MPR of 50%. Standardization of terminology will facilitate health policy decisions based on consistent evidence and ability to appropriately compare and contrast adherence-related studies. Standard terminology will better allow clinicians and investigators to communicate more precisely and accurately.

The term, *nonadherence*, is an overarching statement that by itself does not lead to an appropriate solution. The problem of medication nonadherence is preventable. For many, this is the holy grail of improved quality, and reduced costs in medical care is a desirable mission.

Primary nonadherence occurs when the patient never fills a prescription or never initially begins a medication. Secondary nonadherence occurs when a patient starts the medication for some time but later becomes nonadherent. Another approach to understanding adherence is to differentiate between intentional versus unintentional nonadherence. Clearly, intervening with unintentional nonadherence would appear to be more impactful.

Adherence also has a high intraindividual complex variability; for example, a patient may be adherent to a lipid-lowering regimen but not to the diabetes protocol. In 6 months' time, however, the reverse may be true. Thus, a nonadherent behavior may be disease dependent and also time dependent.

ADHERENCE IN DIABETES

Evidence has linked better medication adherence in diabetes patients with lower total health care costs, including lower hospitalization rates. In a recent report from Vanderbilt University, subjects with diabetes reported family members' nonsupportive behaviors, which were associated with being less adherent to the diabetes medication regimen. Nonsupportive family behaviors sabotaged the subjects' efforts to perform the recommended behaviors. Family members can help an affected individual's motivation to self-manage diabetes.

Nonadherence and nonpersistence to prescribed T2DM medications are, however, common and remain a barrier to optimal health outcomes.[12] A recent meta-analysis of 27 studies of adherence rates to T2DM medications found that only 22% of studies reported greater than or equal to 80% adherence among patients.[13] A systematic review of observational studies reporting persistence with oral antidiabetic drugs (OADs) in patients with T2DM revealed a mean rate of 56.2%, with discontinuation estimates of 31.4%. Similarly, using claims data, rates of insulin glargine persistence in the first year after initiation of approximately 55.0% were reported.[14] The reasons for T2DM medication nonadherence and nonpersistence are multifactorial and include suboptimal communication between patients and providers, inadequate patient knowledge about medications, complex regimens and follow-up, and unique issues surrounding injectables, including insulin.[15]

Many people with diabetes also experience problems due to medication costs, and asking patients about their ability to afford treatment is important. Comorbid chronic illness (eg, depression and chronic pain) as well as more general psychosocial problems can pose significant barriers to diabetes self-management; identifying and rectifying these issues may help improve drug adherence.

There also is evidence that nonadherence and nonpersistence are linked to regimen complexity in chronic diseases, including DM.[16] The Global Attitudes of Patients and Physicians in Insulin Therapy study indicates that number of insulin injections and requirements for dosing at specific times are among the most commonly reported difficulties associated with insulin therapy.[17]

ADHERENCE DATA IN OLDER ADULTS

There is a high prevalence of nonadherence among older adults[18] with T2DM.[19] This may in part be due to the medical team communicating in a generic way with older adults rather than individualizing the recommendations. In a study from University of Chicago, a majority of older patients expressed their health care goals in a social and functional language, rather than the biomedical language used by the medical team.[19] Patients' predominant health care goals centered on maintaining their independence and their activities of daily living (71%). Medical experiences of friends and family (50%), social comparison with peers (7%), and medical professionals (43%) shaped patients' goals. Self-reported medication adherence and glucose monitoring were high, but more than one-quarter of patients failed to adhere to any dietary recommendations, and one-third failed to adhere to their exercise regimens. These results emphasize the importance of patient-centricity in the care of older individuals with diabetes.

There appear to be low levels of adherence to treatment recommendations across health states, treatments, and ages. As many as 60% of persons with chronic disorders are poorly adherent to treatment and in a meta-analysis of medication nonadherence rates in the elderly, it was shown that close to 30% to 60% of outpatients do not take medications as prescribed.[20] On average, only half the patients achieve a therapeutic effect. This lack of benefit may lead to further nonadherence. In the meantime, the chronic condition may worsen. For example, for congestive heart failure, treatment failure or inadequate treatment is the most common cause of hospitalization in people over age 65.

Underdosing also may cause treatment outcomes to vary when a patient is discharged from the hospital. Adherence rates plummet from nearly 100% in the inpatient setting to 60% or less at home and this nonadherence leads to hospital readmissions from 5% to 40% of the time.[21]

Why do individuals miss dosing events? The most common reason given by patients for missing medication is forgetting. A second reason includes symptom management, that is, more medication than prescribed may be taken in the face of increased symptoms while less medication may be taken in the presence of side effects or lack of symptoms. Schedule disruptions form a third reason for missed dosing events.[22] These include factors, such as travel, dining out, interruptions, and so on. Once patients have made a decision to adopt a regimen, the poor adherence problems appear to be pragmatic ones rather than motivational.

Age, however, when examined in the older adult group, is a demographic attribute shown to predict levels of adherence.[23] Adherence has been found particularly problematic for the old-old, or those over 75. The age differences in medication adherence are believed to be mediated by cognitive changes. The young-old, or those 60 years to 70 years old, demonstrate the highest levels of adherence, whereas the adherence levels of those over age 75 are the lowest. This age group, as well as their young-old counterparts, have several critical factors associated with cognitive problems, which may influence medication taking The risk factors for cognitive impairments in those over 65 years of age are (1) the aging neurologic system and cognitive changes related to aging; (2) the existence of 1 or multiple chronic illnesses, which may have an impact on cognition; (3) this age group prescribed multiple prescription medications; and (4) the related higher than normal incidence of side effects, including cognitive side effects, of medication (**Table 1**). Thus, when addressing the older adult population, attention to age category may be important.

A recent systematic analysis[24] examining adherence in older adults found 80 factors related to reduced adherence, which can be categorized into 5 groups: patient factors, health care provider factors, health system factors, medication attributes, and other factors. Poor communication, lack of patient involvement, and lack of medication review can lead to lack of confidence and trust in the health care team, further aggravating adherence rates. Health care system factors, adversely affecting adherence include lack of patient education, lack of follow-up, lack of a medication schedule, and lack of community services.[25]

IMPACT OF NONADHERENCE ON HEALTH CARE

In patients with diabetes, nonadherence to the treatment leads to multiple adverse outcomes, at the individual level as well as in health care utilization.[26]

Meanwhile, research has set the price tag for the direct costs of medication nonadherence in the United States at more than $100 billion. The Network for Excellence in Health Innovation estimates that nonadherence along with suboptimal prescribing, drug administration, and diagnosis costs the health care system as much as $290 billion per year—or 13% of total health care expenditures.[27]

Determination of the economic burden of chronic diseases involves evaluation of the patients' total medical costs and distinguishing between expected and unexpected costs.[28] Expected costs would be toward outpatient care, medications, tests, and monitoring whereas unexpected costs potentially are avoidable and associated with hospitalizations or emergency room visits. Better medication adherence and persistence resulted in lower unexpected costs with a variety of therapeutic approaches (insulin and/or OADs) and patient populations. As expected, improved adherence was associated with increased pharmacy costs but with off-setting reduced hospitalization costs. Rarely, total health care costs were higher in adherent or persistent patients.

In 1 study, clinical and economic outcomes were examined in a large national cohort of patients (n = 135,639) identified from a US managed care company database.[29] In patients whose adherence level increased (change in MPR from <0.80 to ≥0.80 during follow-up), the risk of hospitalization or emergency room visits declined by 13% to realize national annual cost savings of $4.68 billion annually. It was estimated that eliminating loss of adherence (which occurred in 25% of the patient sample) would lead to an additional saving of $3.61 billion.

Boye and colleagues[30] recently published an analysis of the associations between adherence (MPR and PDC) to glucose-lowering agents and outcomes in older T2DM patients (≥65 years), an important population to study given that the rate of DM in this

Table 1
Barriers to medication adherence in older adults

Barrier	Manifestation of Nonadherence			
	Primary	Secondary	Intentional	Nonintentional
Lack of understanding of disease	X	—	X	—
Lack of self-efficacy	X	—	—	X
Side effects of medication	—	X	X	—
Cost of medication (copayments, direct cost)	X	X	X	—
Complex dosing	X	X	—	X
Schedule disruption	—	X	—	—
Polypharmacy	—	X	—	X
Physical dexterity	X	X	—	—
Health illiteracy	X	X	—	X
Inconsistent access to pharmacy	—	X	—	X
Lack of patient engagement	X	X	X	X
Comorbidities: depression, cognitive impairment	X	X	—	X

X denotes the type of non-adherence associated with the various barriers to adherence. *Data from* Dunbar-Jacob J, Mortimer-Stephens M. Treatment adherence in chronic disease. J Clin Epidemiol. 2001;54(12):S57–60; and Yap AF, Thirumoorthy T, Kwan YH. Systematic review of the barriers affecting medication adherence in older adults. Geriatr Gerontol Int. 2016;16(10):1093–101.

group is twice that in the overall adult population. A reduction in outpatient and acute care costs was determined with increasing medication adherence ($10,788 and $18,967, respectively, from least [PDC <20%] to most [PDC ≥80%] adherent patients; P<.005). Consequently, a comparison of the least and most adherent patients was associated with total all-cause cost savings of $28,824 over the 3-year study period. Furthermore, the study estimated savings of $65,464 over 3 years for every 1% increase in adherence per 1000 patients.

There are few data in this area of nonadherence costs from the developing world and from sectors that fall outside of health care budgets, such as social and community care and patient out-of-pocket expenses.[31] Employer costs, absenteeism, and short-term disability costs rarely are included.[32]

Confounding variables in this area include the duration of diabetes and over-reliance on administrative claims data, which may not tell the full story. It is possible that the healthy adherer may be associated with other healthy behaviors, which also would result in improved health outcomes.

SPECIFIC STRATEGIES TO IMPROVE ADHERENCE
Shared Decision Making

Shared decision making is a recommended approach, consisting of 4 components: establishing an ongoing partnership between the provider and the patient, exchange of information regarding risk factors control and currently proved treatment for the condition, deliberation on choices, and making the decision.

Knowing a patient's goal regarding the disease, educational approaches should be made individually. The patient's quality of life and cognitive and functional status all should be included in the management plan.[33] Patients will be informed of the importance of risk factors control to prevent complications so that they can set their goals and priorities according to their needs. There are conditions when family members involve in shared decision making due to patients' cognitive decline or inability to make their own decisions.

Diabetes educators have developed a thoughtful recommendation for enhancing the effectiveness of not only disease education but also improved self-care.[34] It is important to have individualized education based on assessment of an individual's relevant medical history, age, cultural influences, health beliefs and attitudes, diabetes knowledge, self-management skills and behaviors, readiness to learn, health literacy level, physical limitations, family support, and financial status. In addition, functional health literacy level can affect patients' self-management, communication with clinicians, and diabetes outcomes.[35] Simple tools[36] exist for measuring functional health literacy as part of an overall assessment process.

Health Literacy

Common among older adults, low health literacy often is associated with poor adherence.[37] This suggested association implies a need for effective adherence interventions in low health literate people. A previous review,[38] however, show mixed results on the association between low health literacy and poor adherence. A systematic metareview of systematic reviews was conducted to study the association between health literacy and adherence in adults above the age of 50. Evidence for the effectiveness of adherence interventions among adults in this age group with low health literacy also was explored.

Evidence on the association between health literacy and adherence in older adults is relatively weak. Adherence interventions are potentially effective for the vulnerable population of older adults with low levels of health literacy, but the evidence on this topic is limited. Further research is needed on the association between health literacy and general health behavior and on the effectiveness of interventions. It is possible that health literacy is not an independent variable but may not be as critical in those with a very high regard for the health care team and its recommendations; that is, these individuals are less skeptical and have a strong trait of following ritualistic protocols.

Polypill

Polypharmacy is one of the common conditions in older adults when dealing with the health care of these populations. There is no accurate number of medications to define polypharmacy; however, it is commonly accepted as greater than or equal to 5 medications in a patient. Recent data show patients are taking more pills compared with previous decades.[39]

Every medication has its benefits and side effects. Taking more pills simply increases the risk of more side effects. Drug-to-drug interaction is another outcome that can happen, especially if a patient is taking medications that have similar pharmacokinetics. Moreover, aging itself can alter pharmacokinetics and pharmacodynamics of drugs in many ways in older adults, including decreased absorption, metabolism, and excretion.

The complexity of taking multiple medications at various times of the day makes it more likely that a patient omits 1 or more medications. This has led to testing the concept of a polypill (consisting of multiple medications) taken once daily to improve adherence and improve clinical outcomes.

Diabetes is an ideal testing platform, with the need to control multiple metabolic targets for optimal cardiovascular risk reduction. Antihypertensive, lipid-lowering, antidiabetic, and antiplatelet treatments all substantially reduce the risk of cardiovascular events. Recent studies in patients with cardiovascular disease have documented that different cardiovascular drugs can be combined in a single tablet. A recent modeling study based on medication use and adherence data from UnitedHealthcare claims data compared usual care to polypill-based care with 3 versions, using a validated microsimulation model in the National Health and Nutrition Examination Survey population with prior cardiovascular disease. Usual care included individual prescription of up to 4 drug classes (antiplatelet agents, β-blockers, renin-angiotensin-aldosterone inhibitors, and statins). The polypills modeled were aspirin, 81 mg; atenolol, 50 mg; ramipril, 5 mg; and simvastatin, 40 mg (polypill I), atorvastatin, 80 mg (polypill II), or rosuvastatin, 40 mg (polypill III). The incremental cost-effectiveness ratios for polypill I and polypill II were $20,073/quality-adjusted life year and $21,818/quality-adjusted life year , respectively. The study concluded that polypill II model gave the best outcomes whereas polypill I was the cheaper option.[40] All polypills bested usual care.

Despite the anticipated benefits of a polypill, hard evidence that the polypill results in better outcomes than standard individual medication regimens is still awaited.[41,42]

Meanwhile, technology is advancing. Scientists from Europe demonstrated success with a stereolithographic 3-dimensional printing of 6 different medications, with excellent pharmacokinetics.[43] In the future an individualized polypill format that should further enhance adherence can be envisioned.

APPS FOR MEDICATION ADHERENCE

Since patients adhere to only 50% of drugs prescribed for chronic diseases in developed nations and there are not enough clinicians/counselors and time to devote to each individual's nonadherence, digital health has paved the way for innovative smartphone solutions to tackle this challenge.[44] Many mobile apps devoted to medication adherence are available (ie, MyMedSchedule, MyMeds, MedSimple, Med Agenda, PillManager, and RxmindMe). There is a need for evidence of their real-world effectiveness in improving adherence in patients with DM or other chronic diseases.[45] Evidence for the effectiveness of medication reminders using a short message service, or text messaging, in the improvement of DM adherence has, however, been published.[46] This may represent a promising approach because it does not require any extensive investment of health care provider time and easily can be integrated into the daily lives of patients, although its long-term effectiveness currently is unknown.

A recent review of medication adherence apps, examining their development, found that there are thousands of apps available on the Apple App Store and the Google Play Store. Data extracted included app store source, app price, documentation of health care professional (HCP) involvement during app development, and evidence base for each respective app.[47] Free apps were downloaded to explore the strategies used to promote medication adherence. Testing involved a standardized medication regimen of 3 reminders over a 4-hour period. Nonadherence features designed to enhance user experience also were documented.

Of a total of 5881 apps, 805 fulfilled the inclusion criteria initially and were tested. Furthermore, 681 apps were further analyzed for data extraction. Of these, 420 apps were free for testing, 58 were inaccessible, and 203 required payment. Of the 420 free apps, 57 apps were developed with HCP involvement and an evidence base was identified in only 4 apps. Of the paid apps, 9 apps had HCP involvement, 1 app had a documented evidence base, and 1 app had both. In addition, 18 inaccessible apps were produced with HCP involvement, whereas 2 apps had a documented evidence base. The 420 free apps were analyzed further to identify strategies used to improve medication adherence. This identified 3 broad categories of adherence strategies: reminder, behavioral, and educational. A total of 250 apps utilized a single method, 149 apps used 2 methods, and only 22 apps utilized all 3 methods. These data indicate that the end user may have a falsely high level of expectation of app quality and that many of these apps have had little clinical input into their development or weak evidence of effectiveness.

Gamification, using video game elements to better engage patients and improve adherence, is still early in incorporation into adherence solutions, with just 1.2% (5/420) of apps utilizing this technique. One systematic review demonstrated that 69% of psychological therapy outcomes and 59% of physical therapy outcomes were improved by video games; results did not differ across age groups.

Although many of these gamification apps are intended for younger patients, more apps are likely to be developed for older adults. Because nonadherence is common among older adults, it is gratifying to see that their interest in app-based adherence interventions and in mobile health.[48] Enhanced features, such as increased font/text size and a larger keypad, will help increase uptake by older adults.

Recently, the US Food and Drug Administration created a new category of class II integrated continuous glucose monitoring devices and announced new guidelines to accelerate the approval of future products.

INTERVENTIONS FOR ADHERENCE TO ANTI–DIABETES MELLITUS MEDICATIONS

A recent review by Costa and colleagues[5] examined approximately 50 studies of patient-level interventions. Interventions were classified as educational (n = 7), behavioral (n = 3), affective, economic (n = 3), or multifaceted (a combination of the above; n = 40). One study consisted of 2 interventions. Multifaceted interventions, addressing several nonadherence factors, were comparatively more effective in improving medication adherence and glycemic target in patients with T2DM than single strategies. No single intervention was dramatically successful. Educational strategies are the most popular intervention strategy, followed by behavioral, with affective components becoming more common in recent years. Most of the interventions addressed patient-related (n = 35), condition-related (n = 31), and therapy-related (n = 20) factors as defined by the WHO, whereas fewer addressed health care system (n = 5) and socioeconomic-related factors (n = 13).

It is apparent a monotonic approach will not work at improving adherence. Multifaceted symphonic intervention strategies are necessary to have an impact on medication adherence. These strategies need to be personalized, however. Multifocused interventions that include cognitive, behavioral, and affective components demonstrate better outcomes than single approaches.[49]

What can a clinician do to improve adherence?

The Five Es

1. Entry—patient must be able to access the appropriate medications
2. Explain—describe the rationale and simplify the regimen
3. Engage—shared decision making and adapt for health literacy
4. Empower—migration of having the patient be in charge instead of the clinician
5. Encourage—never give up after temporary setbacks; even small improvements can lead to greater changes

FUTURE CONSIDERATIONS

Nonadherence is a form of human behavior, a complex multifactorial phenomenon with great time variation as well as intraindividual variation. It would be analogous to having a lock's combination be constantly changing and thus needing to continuously modify the correct combination to unlock the mechanism. Single component solutions may be easier to implement but are less likely to be successful in the long term.

Adherence solutions must be patient-centric and must be individualized/personalized.[50] In tailoring an intervention, the strategies tend to be more patient centered. More than half of the interventions included in this review considered the individual patient's circumstance(s) while delivering the intervention; however, the extent of individualization varied. Each component (educational, behavioral, affective, or economic) needs to be patient centered. Williams and colleagues[51] also have emphasized the need for tailored interventions to promote medication adherence in patients with T2DM.

Financial or economic factors, such as co-payments, could have an impact on adherence, but, interestingly, adherence is still low in countries where medication access is much better than in the United States. Intervention trials have been inconsistent. Economic incentives will have to be part of the solution and not the only solution to improve adherence in T2DM.

Strategies to improve patient compliance regardless of health issue, theory base, or method yield significant, yet low–moderate effect sizes seldom greater than 0.37 (Dunbar and Mortimer-Stephens). It is likely that this is a function of the multiple determinants of poor adherence episodes.

As a fifth decade of research on patient adherence commences, several issues remain to be addressed. Clearly, more effort needs to be expended on intervention studies. Given the identification of various patterns of missed events and the pragmatic reasons for many of these events, examining intervention strategies targeted to specific problems may be a worthwhile venture. Further exploration of these reasons for missed dosing events would be useful in designing intervention strategies. The major costs of poor adherence also suggest that intervention strategies should be evaluated for their cost-effectiveness. Little attention also has been given to the impact of adherence improvement on clinical outcomes. It would be fruitful to examine the predictors of adherence further, which thus would be useful in targeting subgroups for adherence attention. The newer technologies for assessment and evaluation offer a more sophisticated analysis of adherence behavior.

Improvement in adherence to lifestyle as well as medications will have a huge impact on the cost of diabetes to individuals and to society at large. This will require a multipronged approach, which is flexible and modifiable according to the changing individual needs.

DISCLOSURE

The authors have nothing to disclose.

REFERENCES

1. Bagust A, Hopkinson PK, Maslove L, et al. The projected health care burden of Type 2 diabetes in the UK from 2000 to 2060. Diabetic Med 2002;19:1–5.
2. World Health Organization. World population ageing 2015. Available at: http://www.un.org/en/development/desa/population/publications/pdf/ageing/WPA2015_Report.pdf. Accessed May 7, 2020.
3. Onder G, Bonassi S, Abbatecola AM, et al. Geriatrics Working Group of the Italian Medicines Agency. High prevalence of poor quality drug prescribing in older individuals: a nationwide report from the Italian Medicines Agency (AIFA). J Gerontol A Biol Sci Med Sci 2014;69(4):430–7.
4. Stewart D, Mair A, Wilson M, et al, SIMPATHY consortium. Guidance to manage inappropriate polypharmacy in older people: systematic review and future developments. Expert Opin Drug Saf 2017;16(2):203–13.
5. Costa E, Giardini A, Savin M, et al. Interventional tools to improve medication adherence: review of literature. Patient Prefer Adherence 2015;9:1303.
6. Kaiser family Foundation. Prescription drug Trends. 2019. Available at: https://www.kff.org/tag/prescription-drugs/. Accessed May 7, 2020.
7. Osterberg L, Blaschke T. Adherence to medication. N Engl J Med 2005;353(5):487–97.
8. Lemstra M, Nwankwo C, Bird Y, et al. Primary nonadherence to chronic disease medications: a meta-analysis. Patient Prefer Adherence 2018;12:721.
9. Sabateé E. Adherence to long term therapies: evidence for action. World Health Organization; 2003. Available at: http://apps.who.int/iris/bitstream/10665/42682/1/9241545992.pdf. Accessed November 13, 2019.
10. Cramer JA, Roy A, Burrell A, et al. Medication compliance and persistence: terminology and definitions. Value Health 2008;11(1):44–7.
11. Steiner JF, Prochazka AV. The assessment of refill compliance using pharmacy records. Methods, validity, and applications. J Clin Epidemiol 1997;50:105–16.
12. Polonsky WH, Henry RR. Poor medication adherence in type 2 diabetes: recognizing the scope of the problem and its key contributors. Patient Prefer Adherence 2016;10:1299–307.
13. Sapkota S, Brien JA, Greenfield J, et al. A systematic review of interventions addressing adherence to anti-diabetic medications in patients with type 2 diabetes—impact on adherence. PLoS One 2015;10(2):e0118296.

14. Vrijens B, De Geest S, Hughes DA, et al. A new taxonomy for describing and defining adherence to medications. Br J Clin Pharmacol 2012;73(5):691–705.

15. Gillespie R, Mullan J, Harrison L. Managing medications: the role of informal caregivers of older adults and people living with dementia. A review of the literature. J Clin Nurs 2014;23(23–24):3296–308.

16. Ingersoll KS, Cohen J. The impact of medication regimen factors on adherence to chronic treatment: a review of literature. J Behav Med 2008;31(3):213–24.

17. Peyrot M, Barnett AH, Meneghini LF, et al. Factors associated with injection omission/non-adherence in the global attitudes of patients and Physicians in insulin therapy study. Diabetes Obes Metab 2012;14(12):1081–7.

18. Niehoff KM, Mecca MC, Fried TR. Medication appropriateness criteria for older adults: a narrative review of criteria and supporting studies. Ther Adv Drug Saf 2019;10:1–9.

19. Huang ES, Gorawara-Bhat R, Chin MH. Self reported goals of older patients with type 2 diabetes mellitus. J Am Geriatr Soc 2005;53(2):306–11.

20. Pasina L, Brucato AL, Falcone C, et al. Medication non-adherence among elderly patients newly discharged and receiving polypharmacy. Drugs Aging 2014; 31(4):283–9.

21. Sullivan SD. Noncompliance with medication regimens and subsequent hospitalization: a literature analysis and cost of hospitalization estimate. J Res Pharm Econ 1990;2:19–33.

22. Graveley EA, Oseasohn CS. Multiple drug regimens: medication compliance among veterans 65 years and older. Res Nurs Health 1991;14(1):51–8.

23. Park DC, Willis SL, Morrow D, et al. Cognitive function and medication usage in older adults. J Appl Gerontol 1994;13(1):39–57.

24. Yap AF, Thirumoorthy T, Kwan YH. Systematic review of the barriers affecting medication adherence in older adults. Geriatr Gerontol Int 2016;16(10): 1093–101.

25. Yap AF, Thirumoorthy T, Kwan YH. Medication adherence in the elderly. J Clin Gerontol Geriatr 2016;7(2):64–7.

26. Ho PM, Rumsfeld JS, Masoudi FA, et al. Effect of medication nonadherence on hospitalization and mortality among patients with diabetes mellitus. Arch Intern Med 2006;166(17):1836–41.

27. NEHI. How many more studies will it take? A collection of evidence that our health care system can do better. 2008. Available at: http://www.nehi.net/publications/ 30/how_many_more_studies_will_it_take. Last. Accessed October 15, 2011.

28. Ascher-Svanum H, Lage MJ, Perez-Nieves M, et al. Early discontinuation and restart of insulin in the treatment of type 2 diabetes mellitus. Diabetes Ther 2014;5(1):225–42.

29. Jha AK, Aubert RE, Yao J, et al. Greater adherence to diabetes drugs is linked to less hospital use and could save nearly $5 billion annually. Health Aff (Millwood) 2012;31(8):1836–46.

30. Boye KS, Curtis S, Lage M, et al. Associations between adherence and outcomes among older, type 2 diabetes patients: evidence from a Medicare Supplemental database. Patient Prefer Adherence 2016;16:1573–81.

31. Cheng SH, Chen CC, Tseng CH. Does medication adherence lead to lower healthcare expenses for patients with diabetes? Am J Manag Care 2013;19(8):662–70.

32. Hagen SE, Wright DW, Finch R, et al. Impact of compliance to oral hypoglycemic agents on short-term disability costs in an employer population. Popul Health Manag 2014;17(1):35–41.

33. Ratner NL, Davis EB, Lhotka LL, et al. Patient-centered care, diabetes empowerment, and type 2 diabetes medication adherence among American Indian patients. Clin Diabetes 2017;35(5):281–5.

34. Powers MA, Bardsley J, Cypress M, et al. Diabetes self-management education and support in type 2 diabetes: a joint position statement of the American diabetes association, the American association of diabetes educators, and the Academy of Nutrition and Dietetics. Diabetes Educator 2017;43(1):40–53.

35. Shillinger D, Piette J, Grumbach K, et al. Closing the loop: physician communication with diabetic patients who have low health literacy. Arch Intern Med 2003; 163:83–90.

36. Chew LD, Bradley KA, Boyko EJ. Brief questions to identify patients with inadequate health literacy. Fam Med 2006;36:588–94.

37. Geboers B, Brainard JS, Loke YK, et al. The association of health literacy with adherence in older adults, and its role in interventions: a systematic meta-review. BMC Public Health 2015;15(1):903.

38. Loke YK, Hinz I, Wang X, et al. Systematic review of consistency between adherence to cardiovascular or diabetes medication and health literacy in older adults. Annals of Pharmacotherapy 2012;46(6):863–72.

39. Fulton MM, Riley Allen E. Polypharmacy in the elderly: a literature review. J Am Acad Nurse Pract 2005;17(4):123–32.

40. Gaziano TA, Pandya A, Sy S, et al. Modeling the cost effectiveness and budgetary impact of Polypills for secondary prevention of cardiovascular disease in the United States. Am Heart J 2019;214:77–87.

41. Coca A, Agabiti-Rosei E, Cifkova R, et al. The polypill in cardiovascular prevention: evidence Fulton MM, Riley Allen E. Polypharmacy in the elderly: a literature review. J Am Acad Nurse Pract 2005;17(4):123–32.

42. Coca A, Agabiti-Rosei E. Limitations and perspective–position paper of the European Society of Hypertension. J Hypertens 2017;35(8):1546–53.

43. Robles-Martinez P, Xu X, Trenfield SJ, et al. 3D printing of a multi-layered polypill containing six drugs using a novel stereolithographic method. Pharmaceutics 2019;11(6):274.

44. Shah VN, Garg SK. Managing diabetes in the digital age. Clin Diabetes Endocrinol 2015;1(1):16.

45. Dayer L, Heldenbrand S, Anderson P, et al. Smartphone medication adherence apps: potential benefits to patients and providers. J Am Pharm Assoc 2013;53(2):172–81.

46. Vervloet M, Linn AJ, van Weert JCM, et al. The effectiveness of interventions using electronic reminders to improve adherence to chronic medication: a systematic review of the literature. J Am Med Inform Assoc 2012;19(5):696–704.

47. Ahmed I, Ahmad NS, Ali S, et al. Medication adherence apps: review and content analysis. JMIR Mhealth Uhealth 2018;6(3):e62.

48. Zullig LL, Gellad WF, Moaddeb J, et al. Improving diabetes medication adherence: successful, scalable interventions. Patient Prefer Adherence 2015;9:139–49.

49. Dunbar-Jacob J, Mortimer-Stephens M. Treatment adherence in chronic disease. J Clin Epidemiol 2001;54(12):S57–60.

50. Nieuwlaat R, Wilczynski N, Navarro T, et al. Interventions for enhancing medication adherence. Cochrane Database Syst Rev 2014;(11):CD000011.

51. Williams A, Manias E, Walker R. Interventions to improve medication adherence in people with multiple chronic conditions: a systematic review. J Adv Nurs 2008; 63(2):132–43.

Management of Inpatient Hyperglycemia and Diabetes in Older Adults

Georgia M. Davis, MD[a], Kristen DeCarlo, MD[b],
Amisha Wallia, MD, MS[b], Guillermo E. Umpierrez, MD, CDE[a],
Francisco J. Pasquel, MD, MPH[a],*

KEYWORDS

- Diabetes • Older adults • Elderly • Hyperglycemia • Insulin • Incretin • Inpatient
- Hospitalized

KEY POINTS

- Diabetes in older adults is a growing public health concern in the outpatient and inpatient settings.
- Most hospitalized patients with diabetes are older (age >65 years), frail, and have multiple comorbidities.
- A comprehensive geriatric assessment and a team-based approach are recommended to tailor an individualized care plan, with consideration of the patients' personal goals, comorbidities, functional status, life expectancy, and risk of clinically significant hypoglycemia and hyperglycemia.
- Cautious use of insulin therapy is recommended in older adults with risk factors for hypoglycemia, including decreased renal function and poor nutritional status.
- The results of recent clinical trials suggest simplified therapeutic regimens using agents with a lower risk of hypoglycemia are preferable for most patients with mild to moderate hyperglycemia.

INTRODUCTION

More than 450 million people worldwide are living with diabetes, leading to an associated estimated global health care expenditure of $850 billion in 2017.[1] By 2030,

Funding: F.J. Pasquel and G.E. Umpierrez are partially supported by NIH grants (1K23GM128221-01A1 [F.J. Pasquel], UL1TR002378 and 1P30DK111024-01 [G.E. Umpierrez]).
[a] Department of Medicine, Division of Endocrinology, Emory University School of Medicine, 69 Jesse Hill Jr Drive Southeast, Atlanta, GA 30303, USA; [b] Division of Endocrinology, Metabolism and Molecular Medicine, Northwestern University Feinberg School of Medicine, 645 N. Michigan Ave, Chicago, IL 60611, USA
* Corresponding author.
E-mail address: fpasque@emory.edu

Clin Geriatr Med 36 (2020) 491–511
https://doi.org/10.1016/j.cger.2020.04.008
0749-0690/20/© 2020 Elsevier Inc. All rights reserved.

geriatric.theclinics.com

global costs of diabetes are estimated exceed 2015 levels by 88%, accounting for 2.2% of the global gross domestic product (compared with 1.8% in 2015).[2] In addition to the socioeconomic burden on national health care systems and global economies, diabetes disproportionally affects older adults. It is estimated that 1 in 5 individuals older than 65 years has diabetes in the United States.[3] Not only are older individuals more likely to have diabetes, but those with diabetes are 3 times more likely to require hospital admission compared with younger individuals.[4]

Glycemic control in the hospital setting is important for reducing complications and mortality[5–7]; however, maintaining strict or tight glycemic control in the inpatient setting has been associated with poor outcomes related to iatrogenic hypoglycemia.[8] The balance between achieving glycemic control and avoiding hypoglycemia is especially challenging in older individuals with longer diabetes duration, diabetes-related complications, multiple medical comorbidities, and functional decline. It is important to consider the following factors when determining glycemic targets and diabetes treatment regimens in elderly patients, including functional status, life expectancy, level of frailty, and cognitive impairment.

Research focused on inpatient diabetes management in older patients has been limited.[9] We review the prevalence, clinical presentation, and assessment of older adults with diabetes in the hospital. We also explore the role of multidisciplinary team approach, diabetes education, glycemic control strategies, and recommendations for discharge regimens in this population.

PREVALENCE AND ECONOMIC BURDEN

From 2000 to 2010, the prevalence of diabetes in the United States increased from 39% to 42% according to data from the National Inpatient Sample Database.[10] Most of the reported diabetes in older adults is attributed to type 2 diabetes, which is the focus of this review. However, type 1 diabetes has been estimated to account for between 5% and 10% of diabetes cases worldwide, with most cases diagnosed in childhood and young adulthood, although several studies suggest an additional rise in diagnosis rates later in life (age >50 years).[11,12] A total of 7.2 million hospital discharges included diabetes as a hospital diagnosis among US adults in 2014.[13] Between 2007 and 2014 there were more than 32 million hospitalizations of patients with diabetes older than 65 years,[14] representing 57% of all admissions of patients with diabetes. Over the same period, there was also an increase in hospital admissions for hyperglycemic crises (0.8% in 2007 to 1.2% in 2014), with older adults experiencing a disproportionally high mortality rate (12.8%) in this setting.[14]

The total costs of diagnosed diabetes have increased to $327 billion in 2017 from $245 billion in 2012.[15] The continued increase in diabetes costs in the United States is primarily related to the growing diabetes prevalence among the older adult population ≥65 years of age. Approximately 61% of all diabetes health care expenditures are attributed to health resources for older adults.[15] The average annual excess expenditures for those younger than 65 years and older than 65 years is estimated at $6675 and $13,239, respectively. Approximately 30% of total diabetes care costs represent inpatient care.[15]

Hyperglycemia, defined as a blood glucose (BG) >140 mg/dL, commonly occurs in hospitalized older adult patients. Approximately one-third of general medicine and surgery patients older than 65 years develop hyperglycemia during hospital admission, with hyperglycemia rates increasing to more than 70% in critically ill and cardiac surgery patients of similar age.[16–19] In addition, older adults with diabetes have higher hospitalization rates compared to patients without diabetes. Older adults with uncontrolled diabetes (hemoglobin A1c [HbA1c] >7%) have disproportionally higher hospital admission rates compared to those with controlled diabetes, prediabetes, or without a diagnosis of diabetes.[20] The presence of diabetes and hyperglycemia in an aging population is often associated with poor outcomes, highlighting the importance of determining effective inpatient and outpatient treatment regimens.

PATHOPHYSIOLOGY

Aging itself has a complex effect on glucose metabolism, including beta-cell dysfunction, changes in insulin secretion and insulin resistance, as well as fat regulation.[21] A decrease in beta-cell function and insulin secretion is known to occur with aging.[22] The etiology of hyperglycemia and diabetes in older adults is thought to be multifactorial, and includes genetic factors, diet, lifestyle, body composition, and peripheral insulin sensitivity. Studies comparing hepatic glucose production in younger and older adults have been mixed, and appears that hepatic glucose output may not be affected by age as much as by differences in body composition.[21,23–25] Beta-cell function and insulin secretion in older adults have been shown to be decreased, accompanied by worsening insulin resistance compared with younger adults.[26–28] In addition, changes in body fat mass with a reduction in lean muscle mass that occurs with age, as well as adipose tissue dysfunction (a proinflammatory state) increases insulin resistance in older adults.

Acute illness is associated with increased cortisol and catecholamine release, along with gluconeogenesis and decreased peripheral tissue glucose uptake, all contributing to hyperglycemia during stress. Therefore, older adults in the hospital are particularly susceptible to worsening glucose homeostasis.

ASSESSMENT OF OLDER ADULTS WITH DIABETES IN THE INPATIENT SETTING

Diabetes in older adults is accompanied by elevated risk of diabetes complications and, as expected, is associated with an increased incidence and prevalence of geriatric syndromes.[29,30] Geriatric syndromes are multifactorial clinical conditions in older adults; they can greatly impact diabetes self-care, quality of life, and health outcomes (rehospitalization, mortality).[31,32] These include cognitive or psychological impairments, including depression, delirium, and dementia; also more functional disabilities can be present, including falls, malnutrition, and urinary incontinence.[31,33]

These types of geriatric syndromes are highly prevalent in the inpatient setting. A prospective study of hospitalized adults older than 70 years with diabetes reported high rates of cognitive impairment including dementia (27.8%), delirium (21.1%), depression (38.9%), and dependency in activities of daily living (91.1%).[34] Cognitive evaluation with mini-mental status examination found a low number of patients with normal results (12.2%), and a high number of patients who screened positive for dementia (43.8%) without a prior diagnosis.[34]

Care for older adults with diabetes and hyperglycemia requires assessment of comorbid conditions and geriatric syndromes with a comprehensive geriatric assessment (CGA) (**Fig. 1**).[31] The CGA is a multimodal, multidisciplinary evaluation composed of validated screening tools and assessments targeting medical conditions, functional capacity, as well as cognitive, psychological, and social domains for older adults.[33,35] The individual components of the CGA are required by the Centers for Medicare and Medicaid Services, and are typically conducted by primary care physicians.[36] This evaluation specifically aims to identify existing geriatric syndromes to assess risk, while comprehensively reviewing patients' overall health and values.[37,38] In hospitalized and community-dwelling older adults, routine CGA is associated with improved outcomes,

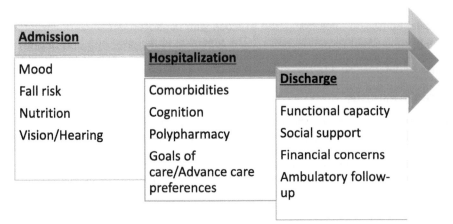

Fig. 1. Comprehensive geriatric assessment throughout the hospital stay.

including lower rates of institutionalization, slower decline in quality of life, and lower mortality rates; it is included in most guidelines for management of diabetes in older adults in both the inpatient and outpatient setting.[30,31,37,39–42]

The CGA can provide a framework for assessment and development of care plans in the inpatient setting. Older adults with diabetes are at risk of progression of such geriatric syndromes.[43] Hospitalization provides an opportunity for the primary team to identify these risks, by careful evaluation of pertinent medical conditions and assessment of cognition, polypharmacy, functional status, and goals of care.[44] The multidisciplinary team for older adults with hyperglycemia/diabetes typically includes (but is not limited to) consultation services (endocrinology, geriatrics, neurology, psychiatry, and palliative care teams), diabetes education, physical and occupational therapy, registered dietitians, pharmacy, nursing, social work, and care management. Using this model, components rather than a full CGA can be best used in the inpatient setting. On discharge, evaluation of functional capacity and social and financial support can help formulate a safe inpatient to outpatient care plan (see **Fig. 1**).

Expert consensus panels have developed targeted geriatric assessment tools; a 1-page assessment specifically based on the CGA was recently validated at a geriatric day hospital in Brazil (mean age 79.5 ± 8.4 years).[45] It included 10 domains (social support, recent hospital admissions, falls, number of medications, activities of daily living, cognitive performance, self-rated health, depressive symptoms, nutritional status, and gait speed).[45] Further, this instrument has been used to predict 1-year mortality in hospitalized older adults (mean age 79.4 ± 8.4 years).[46] This screening tool requires additional testing to validate its widespread use, as efficient CGA models are essential for hospital practice.

Two specific domains, cognitive impairment and frailty, may be most beneficial to assess in a targeted CGA for hospitalized older adults with diabetes. Cognitive impairment is seen in up to half of all older adults with diabetes and is associated with increased risk of hypoglycemia.[47] The validated mini-cog test is used for screening cognitive impairment in older adults in the outpatient setting, taking only approximately 3 minutes to perform.[48,49] Diabetes in older adults is associated with reduced muscle strength, sarcopenia, accelerated loss of muscle mass, and poor muscle quality and represents an independent risk factor for frailty, which, in turn, is associated with increased mortality.[41,50,51] Several frailty-screening tools have been validated and can be used in older adults with diabetes, but there is currently no inpatient gold standard for their use.[52–55]

Multidisciplinary CGA offered in an inpatient geriatric evaluation and management unit, may be beneficial for the care for frail older persons admitted to the hospital and lead to less functional decline at discharge and a lower rate of institutionalization 1-year post discharge.[43] Another successful program is the Acute Care for Elders (ACE) model, developed to prevent functional decline and adverse outcomes after hospitalization in older adults. It is characterized by patient-centered care, and includes frequent medical review, early rehabilitation, and discharge planning. A systematic review and meta-analysis of older adults (average age 81 years) admitted to ACE units (N = 6839) demonstrated fewer falls, less delirium, less functional decline, shorter length of stay, fewer discharges to nursing home, and more discharged to home.[56] These inpatient models highlight the significance of a multidisciplinary team approach and use of the CGA as components of specialized inpatient care for older adults and may play a significant role in care of older adults with diabetes.

MULTIDISCIPLINARY TEAMS AND DIABETES EDUCATION IN OLDER ADULTS

Hospitalization offers a unique opportunity for multidisciplinary care in diabetes management and education with specialty services available if needed (**Fig. 2**). Retrospective studies highlight the significance of specialized diabetes consultation team participation in inpatient glucose management, as demonstrated by reduction in

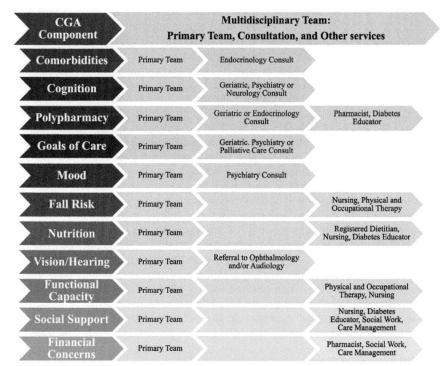

Fig. 2. Components of a comprehensive geriatric assessment (CGA). (*From* DeCarlo K, Wallia A. Inpatient management of T2DM and hyperglycemia in older adults. Curr Diab Rep. 2019;19(10):104; with permission.)

30-day readmission rates and length of stay.[57,58] In addition, formal diabetes education in hospitalized patients with poorly-controlled diabetes is independently associated with lower frequency of hospital readmission at 30 days.[59] A study evaluating the role of a multidisciplinary team focused on inpatient glycemic control, diabetes education, and discharge planning showed improved glycemic control at 1-year post discharge with significant improvement in glycemic control in patients newly started on insulin with an average HbA1c reduction of 2.4%.[60] A multidisciplinary team approach with an individualized diabetes care plan in older adults provides the initial framework for successful long-term diabetes care in this high-risk population.

GLYCEMIC TARGETS

Data from observational studies have shown a consistent association between both hypoglycemia and hyperglycemia with increased complications and mortality in hospitalized patients.[61,62] Although clinical trials in the hospital have included a broad range of participants including older patients, the most frail and elderly populations have often been excluded from these trials.[7,63–65]

Recommendations for glycemic targets in hospitalized patients have historically been divided between populations with critical versus non-critical illness. Even though older adults have been included in these trials, no specific recommendations have been made regarding glycemic target goals based on age and age-related factors alone. In the absence of specific recommendations for inpatient glycemic targets in older adults, we recommend following general clinical guidelines for adult patients, but with an emphasis on hypoglycemia prevention.

The 2019 American Diabetes Association Standards of Medical Care in Diabetes on inpatient glycemic control recommends targeting glucose levels between 140 and 180 mg/dL (7.8–10 mmol/L) for most hospitalized patients (in both critical and non-critical care settings) to improve outcomes associated with uncontrolled hyperglycemia while minimizing the risk of hypoglycemia.[66] Treatment of inpatient hyperglycemia in those with and without diabetes is typically recommended once glucose levels reach 180 mg/dL, including in surgical patients during the perioperative period.[66,67] More stringent goals may be appropriate for select hospital populations (ie, cardiac surgery, acute stroke), provided the targets can be achieved without significant hypoglycemia. However, in agreement with less aggressive glycemic targets, two recent randomized controlled trials (RCTs) in cardiac surgery patients failed to demonstrate that intensive insulin therapy targeting glucose levels between 100 and 140 mg/dL reduced hospital complications when compared with a target glucose range of 140 to 180 mg/dL.[68,69]

Admission HbA1c concentration is a good predictor of inpatient glycemic control and hypoglycemia risk in insulin-treated patients with type 2 diabetes.[70] Patients with admission HbA1c levels less than 7% are more likely to achieve target glucose control during admission, compared with those with HbA1c levels between 7% and 9% and more than 9%, but are also at higher odds for hypoglycemia.[70] To decrease the risk of iatrogenic hypoglycemia, it has been recommended that daily insulin dosage adjustments occur when glucose values fall below 100 mg/dL (5.6 mmol/L).[71] Less stringent target glucose ranges are needed to reduce the risk of hypoglycemia in terminally ill patients, in patients with severe comorbidities, and in care settings in which frequent glucose monitoring or close nursing supervision is not feasible.

INPATIENT HYPOGLYCEMIA

Patients most likely to develop hypoglycemia during admission tend to be older, have more comorbidities, and are receiving insulin therapy.[72] The most common risk factor for inpatient hypoglycemia is treatment with insulin, although other risk factors include use of sulfonylureas, insulin administration errors, poor nutritional intake, and changes to hospital routine.[72–74] Elderly people are also more prone to hypoglycemia due to a higher rate of comorbidities, such as renal failure, malnutrition, malignancies, dementia, and frailty.[75,76]

Several observational and clinical trials have reported that hypoglycemia in hospitalized older adults is associated with longer length of hospital stay and higher mortality.[75,77,78] A case-control study showed that older patients admitted to acute medical and geriatric wards with hypoglycemia had 3.7 higher odds of dying in the hospital. This association was independent from other risk factors.[77] Kagansky and colleagues,[75] in a study including more than 5000 hospitalized patients 70 years or older, found that sepsis, albumin level, malignancy, sulfonylurea and insulin treatment, alkaline phosphatase level, female sex, and creatinine level were all independent predictors of hypoglycemia in the hospital. Hypoglycemia was associated with mortality; however, this association was lost after adjusting for multiple covariates.[75] Additional studies have suggested that in patients with and without diabetes, mortality is associated with spontaneous hypoglycemia and not with iatrogenic hypoglycemia (ie, insulin therapy).[72,79,80] Establishing an independent causal relationship between hypoglycemia and mortality among elderly individuals with multiple comorbidities is complex in observational studies. Clinical trials in non–intensive care unit (ICU) settings have reported an incidence of hypoglycemia of approximately 12% to 38% for patients with type 2 diabetes receiving insulin therapy.[7,64,65,81–83] These trials, however, have reported a very low incidence of severe hypoglycemia in a controlled setting and have not been powered to assess mortality. However, in critically ill patients, the presence and degree of hypoglycemia are related to increasing mortality risk. The Normoglycemia in Intensive Care Evaluation–Survival Using Glucose Algorithm Regulation (NICE-SUGAR) trial reported a mortality rate of 35.4% in those experiencing severe hypoglycemia (<40 mg/dL [2.2 mmol/L]) with an associated hazard ratio for death of 3.21 (95% confidence interval 2.49–4.15) compared to patients without hypoglycemia.[8]

MANAGEMENT OF HYPERGLYCEMIA IN THE INTENSIVE CARE UNIT

Intravenous insulin is the preferred method for treatment of hyperglycemia in the critical care setting, including in older adults. Various continuous insulin infusion protocols for the treatment of medical and surgical ICU patients have been reported in the literature,[84] and more recently computer-based algorithms to guide clinical staff in adjusting insulin infusion have become commercially available. Although the use of computer-based algorithms has been associated with lower rates of hypoglycemia, glycemic variability, and a higher percentage of glucose readings within target range, no studies have evaluated their impact on hospital complications or mortality compared with use of standard paper-based algorithms.[5,85]

MANAGEMENT OF HYPERGLYCEMIA IN NON–CRITICAL CARE SETTINGS
Basal and Rapid-Acting Subcutaneous Insulin

Subcutaneous insulin has been considered the preferred agent for glycemic control in non-ICU settings, typically using basal insulin alone, or in combination with prandial insulin.[71] Selecting insulin treatment regimens in older adult patients offers more complexity related to medical comorbidities, variable nutrition status, or presence of frailty, as well as the associated hypoglycemia risk with increased potential for hypoglycemia unawareness.

For most older adult patients with adequate oral intake and uncontrolled hyperglycemia, a basal-bolus insulin approach may be considered using a starting total daily dose (TDD) of 0.2 to 0.3 units/kg per day, with half of the TDD given as basal insulin and the other half as rapid-acting insulin divided between meals.[9] Variable nutritional status and oral intake may be a more common chronic issue compounded by the effects of acute illness in an older adult population, leading to an increased risk of iatrogenic hypoglycemia with certain insulin regimens. Several studies have shown higher rates of hypoglycemia with use of human insulin (NPH and Regular), particularly with premixed formulations (threefold increase in hypoglycemia) in older adults compared with treatment with a basal-bolus regimen using insulin analogs.[83,86] We recommend against the use of premixed insulin in the hospital.

Several modifications to insulin regimens have been suggested to reduce hypoglycemia in at-risk populations. The Basal Plus[65] trial evaluated treatment with basal and prandial insulin (basal-bolus regimen) compared with basal insulin with only sliding scale insulin (SSI) at mealtimes (basal-plus regimen) or SSI alone in patients with type 2 diabetes. The TDD of insulin was reduced for those with age $\geq$70 years and/or serum creatinine $\geq$2.0 mg/dL with a starting basal dose of 0.15 units/kg per day. Results showed comparable glycemic control and frequency of hypoglycemia between the basal-bolus and basal-plus groups, suggesting that the use of basal insulin with SSI at meals combined with a lower TDD of insulin may be preferred in older patients with poor oral intake.[65] A retrospective study evaluating use of the GesTIO hospital insulin protocol (lower TDD of insulin at 0.2–0.3 units/kg per day and reduction of prandial insulin dose for premeal BG 70–90 mg/dL) in older frail patients showed improvement in mean daily BG, a 9.1% incidence of mild hypoglycemia and no severe episodes of hypoglycemia.[87]

Supplemental/Correction Doses of Short-Acting Insulin ("Sliding Scale")

The use of SSI, regular or rapid-acting insulin administered at scheduled intervals, continues to be a common method for treatment of hyperglycemia in the hospital, including in older patients. The reactive nature of SSI use alone to correct hyperglycemia often predisposes patients to wide glycemic variability with episodes of both hyperglycemia and hypoglycemia, as well as increased risk of complications,[7,64] although some patients with mild hyperglycemia may achieve adequate glycemic control with the use of SSI alone.

INPATIENT USE OF NON-INSULIN THERAPIES FOR MANAGEMENT OF HYPERGLYCEMIA

Due to concerns regarding the safe use of older oral agents in the acute setting, professional associations have recommended the use of insulin regimens as the preferred approach to treat hyperglycemia in the hospital. Safety concerns have been related mainly to the fear of lactic acidosis with metformin, delayed onset of action and volume retention with thiazolidinediones, and sustained hypoglycemia with sulfonylureas.[71,88] Despite such recommendations, the use of oral antidiabetic agents (OADs) is common in clinical practice in the United States and worldwide.[88] No studies, however, have been conducted to prospectively evaluate the safety and efficacy of older OADs in the hospital. In an RCT enrolling residents at long-term care (LTC) or skilled nursing facilities, we observed that the continuation of OADs resulted in similar glycemic control compared with low-dose insulin therapy (glargine, starting dose 0.1 units/kg per day).[89] Nevertheless, a high rate of hypoglycemia was observed in both groups ($\sim$30% of patients over a 26-week period).[89]

More recently, agents associated with a low risk of hypoglycemia (ie, incretin-based therapies) have been prospectively tested in hospitalized patients (including older adults) with diabetes and residents in LTC and skilled nursing facilites.[88,90,91]

INCRETIN-BASED THERAPIES

Incretin agents provide a normal physiologic response in the presence of glucose with a low risk of hypoglycemia.[92,93] Large cardiovascular outcomes trials (CVOTs) testing Dipeptidylpeptidase-4 (DPP-4) inhibitors have confirmed a safe cardiovascular risk profile for this drug class. CVOTs have also confirmed the safety of glucagon-like peptide-1 receptor agonists (GLP-1 RAs) and have reported a reduction in major cardiovascular events.[94–97] In the inpatient setting, clinical trials with DPP-4 inhibitors, native GLP-1, and GLP-1 RAs have shown promising results in acutely ill patients.

Dipeptidylpeptidase-4 Inhibitors

Multiple RCTs and observational studies have reported that DPP-4 inhibitors alone or in combination with basal insulin are safe and effective for the management of general medicine and surgery patients with type 2 diabetes.[98–102] An initial pilot study suggested sitagliptin alone or in combination with basal insulin was effective in patients with type 2 diabetes with mild to moderate hyperglycemia.[99] This study included participants treated at home with diet alone, oral agents, or low doses of insulin (<0.4 units/kg per day). Ninety participants were randomized to sitagliptin, sitagliptin plus basal insulin, or basal-bolus insulin. No differences were observed in the primary outcome of mean daily BG between groups. The TDD of insulin and the number of insulin injections were lower in those receiving sitagliptin. A subanalysis showed, however, that patients with randomization BG >180 mg/dL assigned to sitagliptin alone had higher mean daily BG, suggesting monotherapy with a DPP-4 inhibitor may not be as effective for patients with moderate to severe hyperglycemia. A larger follow up study compared sitagliptin with a single dose of basal insulin with a basal-bolus regimen in a broad population of hospitalized patients with home insulin doses up to 0.6 units/kg per day.[98] Both groups achieved similar glycemic control. Treatment failure occurred in 16% of patients assigned to sitagliptin-basal and 19% of those receiving basal-bolus. Treatment failure was independent of group assignment but was associated with higher A1c levels, as previously described.[70] The odds of treatment failure were 30% higher per 1-unit change in HbA1c (odds ratio 1.3, 95% confidence interval 1.2 -1.5).

In an RCT enrolling only surgical patients, we compared linagliptin versus basal-bolus in patients treated with diet, oral agents, or total insulin dose (TDD) ≤0.5 units/kg per day before admission.[102] We observed a mean daily BG difference of 10.8 mg/dL (95% confidence interval 0.72–22 mg/dL). Among participants with randomization BG <200 mg/dL (63% of cohort), glycemic control was similar in linagliptin and basal-bolus groups (160 ± 41 vs 157 ± 41 mg/dL, $P = .43$); however, patients with BG ≥200 mg/dL assigned to linagliptin had worse glycemic control compared with basal-bolus (196 ± 47 vs 165 ± 47 mg/dL, $P < .001$). Linagliptin resulted in a remarkable reduction in the incidence of hypoglycemic events (1.6% vs 11%, $P = .001$, 86% relative risk reduction). Similarly, Garg and colleagues[101] compared the use of saxagliptin with a basal-bolus regimen and observed no difference in glycemic control in patients with very mild hyperglycemia (admission BG ~150 mg/dL and mean A1c <7%).

In addition, we recently reported the results of an RCT comparing linagliptin with low dose basal insulin in residents of LTC and skilled nursing facilities.[91] Participants had a known history of type 2 diabetes, BG >180 mg/dL, and/or HbA1c >7.5% while receiving treatment with diet, OADs, or insulin at a TDD ≤0.1 units/kg per day. Treatment with linagliptin resulted in noninferior glycemic control compared with insulin glargine. Furthermore, linagliptin resulted in fewer hypoglycemic events less than 70 mg/dL (3% vs 37%) or less than 54 mg/dL (7% vs 0%) compared with glargine.[91] These findings cannot necessarily be translated to the hospital setting; however, they clearly show insulin use in frail patients is associated with a high rate of hypoglycemia even at very low doses.

The results of these trials indicate that treatment with DPP-4 inhibitors is associated with lower rates of hypoglycemia and similar glycemic control compared with more complex insulin regimens, particularly among patients with mild to moderate hyperglycemia (**Fig. 3**).

Glucagon-like Peptide-1 Receptor Agonists

Pilot studies have reported that infusion of native GLP-1 or use of GLP-1 RAs may lead to improved endothelial function,[103] reduced infarct size following myocardial infarction,[104] and increased left ventricular function.[105–108] GLP-1 RA and native GLP-1 have also been tested in critically ill and surgical patients.[109–112] A nonrandomized study in cardiac surgery patients with hyperglycemia suggested intravenous exenatide was effective, and associated with a low risk of hypoglycemia compared with historical controls.[109] Similarly, in a randomized trial, Besch and colleagues[113] reported 72% of patients treated with exenatide and 80% of the insulin-treated group (P = .3) met target glucose concentration. Subjects in the exenatide group received less insulin overall and had a longer time interval to initiation of insulin.

Perioperative treatment with liraglutide, administered before noncardiac surgery, was compared with insulin infusion, or subcutaneous insulin with 50% of home insulin dose given the morning of surgery.[111] Treatment with liraglutide was associated with lower glucose levels 1 hour after surgery with no differences in hypoglycemia or postoperative complications. Liraglutide use was associated with increased preoperative

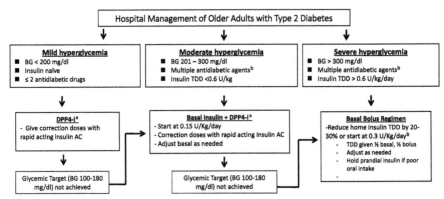

Fig. 3. Recommendations to start antihyperglycemic therapy in older adults with type 2 diabetes in the hospital. No prospective studies have determined the efficacy of other oral antidiabetic drugs in the hospital setting. AC, before meals; TDD, total daily dose. [a] Adjust dose according to GFR (sitagliptin or saxagliptin), no adjustment is needed with linagliptin. [b] Antidiabetic agents: oral agents and GLP-1 RA. (*Adapted from* Pasquel FJ, Fayfman M, Umpierrez GE. Debate on insulin vs non-insulin use in the hospital setting-is it time to revise the guidelines for the management of inpatient diabetes? Curr Diab Rep. 2019;19(9):65; with permission.)

nausea rates. Similarly, preliminary results of the GLOBE trial[114] presented at the American Diabetes Association Scientific Sessions in 2019, showed that liraglutide administered before surgery resulted in significant improvement in glycemic control with lower insulin requirements after cardiac surgery.[115]

We recently compared subcutaneous exenatide 5 µg administered twice daily both with and without basal insulin with a standard basal-bolus insulin regimen in general medicine and surgery patients with diabetes.[116] Patients receiving exenatide plus basal insulin in the hospital achieved similar mean BG compared with those on basal-bolus insulin (154 ± 39 vs 166 ± 40 mg/dL, $P = .31$) and lower mean BG compared with exenatide treatment alone (177 ± 4 mg/dL, $P = .02$). A higher proportion of participants in the exenatide plus basal insulin group had BG readings within target range of 70 to 180 mg/dL (78%) compared with exenatide alone (62%) or basal-bolus insulin (63%). Patients receiving exenatide experienced higher rates of nausea.[116]

These studies suggest GLP-1 RA may be efficacious in controlling glucose levels without increasing the risk of hypoglycemia. Its use, however, may be limited by potential risk of gastrointestinal side effects and may need to be avoided in people who have active gastrointestinal conditions or those who are frail and have poor oral intake.

We conducted a pooled analysis of incretin-based therapies in inpatient older adults with type 2 diabetes, including a total of 192 elderly patients treated incretin therapy (DPP-4 inhibitor or GLP-1 RA) alone, incretin therapy plus basal with insulin, or basal-bolus. Incretin therapy was associated with similar glycemic control and lower rates of hypoglycemia compared with a complex basal-bolus regimen.[117]

SODIUM GLUCOSE CO-TRANSPORTER-2 INHIBITORS

Sodium glucose co-transporter-2 (SGLT-2) inhibitors are a class of oral antihyperglycemic agents that prevent glucose reabsorption by the kidneys leading to glycosuria.[118] In addition to improving glycemic control, large CVOTs have shown that SGLT-2 inhibitors have significant cardiovascular benefit, with large RCTs showing reduced cardiovascular disease–related mortality, fewer hospitalizations for heart failure, as well as a reduction in renal outcomes in patients with diabetic kidney disease.[119–121] These cardiorenal outcomes have also been observed in older adults.[122] Despite these benefits, SGLT-2 inhibitors can lead to side effects that may limit their potential for use in the hospital, such as euglycemic diabetic ketoacidosis, acute kidney injury, volume depletion, and genitourinary infections. These potential side effects make the use of SGLT-2 inhibitors less attractive in older patients with acute illnesses requiring hospitalizations.

ADVANCES IN DIABETES TECHNOLOGY IN THE HOSPITAL

The use of diabetes technology is emerging in the inpatient setting and includes the use of continuous glucose monitoring (CGM) and insulin pump technology. CGM has allowed for more complete characterization of glycemic control by providing estimated BG values every 5 to 15 minutes using a small subcutaneous sensor. Although CGM use in the hospital remains investigational, a recent pilot study explored its use in an older adult population to alert nursing staff to hypoglycemic events.[123] Patients were randomized to standard-of-care capillary glucose monitoring versus real-time CGM with data transmitted to nursing personnel in a telemetry-type method with an alert for sensor glucose values 85 mg/dL or lower. In this study, overall rates of hypoglycemia were lower in the intervention group, and no patient in this group experienced severe hypoglycemia. This study supports continued research into use of CGM for prevention of hypoglycemia in older adult patients with risk factors for hypoglycemia and hypoglycemia unawareness.

Leading edge diabetes technology also includes the use of hybrid closed-loop, or artificial pancreas technology. This refers to the use of CGM and insulin pump therapy integrated with an algorithm for insulin infusion adjustments based on CGM glucose values. A recent study investigated the use of hybrid closed-loop therapy compared with standard basal-bolus insulin administration in non–critically ill hospitalized patients with type 2 diabetes (mean age 67 years).[124] Time in target glucose range (100–180 mg/dL) was higher in the closed-loop group compared with conventional insulin therapy ($65.8 \pm 16.8\%$ vs $41.5 \pm 16.9\%$, $P < .001$) without increased rates of hypoglycemia. Further studies are needed to assess feasibility, patient-centered outcomes, and cost-effectiveness of hybrid closed-loop therapy, especially in an older adult inpatient population.

DISCHARGE PLANNING

Hospital hyperglycemia management is anchored on insulin therapy; however, not all patients require the same home regimen. Discharge for older adults can be clinically complex, given comorbidities, complex drug regimens, and assessment of geriatric needs (such as the components of the comprehensive geriatric assessment). The Endocrine Society recently published guidelines for the care of diabetes in older adults in which a tiered framework was reviewed to categorize patients by level of health and mortality risk. In categorizing healthy, intermediate health, and poor health by evaluation of chronic conditions, visual impairment, and functional status, one can appropriately recommend goals of care.[37,125] It is recommended that the outpatient goal HbA1c for healthy elderly patients to be 7.0% to 7.5%, intermediate health group 7.5% to 8.0%, and those with poor health 8.0% to 8.5%.[37]

Although inpatient or recent HbA1c can help guide discharge therapy, there have been no validated algorithms or studies evaluating discharge recommendations in older adults only. However, we have previously recommended the following discharge diabetes therapy in older adults: admission HbA1c range < 7.5% to 8%, restart home regimen (oral agents with insulin if necessary); HbA1c 8.0% to 10.0%, consider oral agents plus basal insulin (50% of hospital basal insulin dose); and for HbA1c >10%, patients should be discharged on a basal-bolus insulin regimen or on a combination of preadmission oral agents with approximately 80% of hospital basal insulin dose[9]; this is less aggressive than our treatment algorithm in a broad inpatient population.[126] It is prudent to evaluate at discharge the ability of a patient to perform self-care, such as glucose monitoring, ability to self-inject, and oral intake and/or ability to complete activities of daily living. Based on this assessment, the diabetes plan may need to be tailored to include modified regimens (eg, use of long-acting insulin with other non-insulin agents) or utilization of caregivers to help with diabetes self-care.

In the outpatient setting, simplifying insulin regimens can be markedly beneficial in this population. Munshi and colleagues[127] noted a reduction in hypoglycemia and diabetes-related distress, without an associated change in HbA1c with simplification of insulin regimens. Modifications for simplification included moving bedtime basal insulin injections to morning, changing from pre-mixed to basal insulin formulations, and reducing and/or switching prandial insulin in combination with oral medications.

Metformin should be considered a first-line agent at discharge, assuming no contraindications (severe renal disease, gastrointestinal distress). DPP-4 inhibitors have been shown to be safe and efficacious in older adults with less adverse events compared with sulfonylureas.[128] A recent RCT showed a twofold increase in the probability of achieving glycemic targets without an excess of hypoglycemia after adding a DPP-4 inhibitor in older patients treated with basal insulin.[129] The addition of sitagliptin and metformin at discharge following an HbA1c-based algorithm was efficacious in a broad inpatient population.[130] We suggest caution when adding new OADs to older adults treated with insulin or sulfonylureas. A careful reduction in insulin doses or discontinuation of sulfonylureas (particularly glyburide) when replacing with agents with low risk of hypoglycemia is recommended. More data have been forthcoming on the safety and use of SGLT-2 inhibitors in older adults.[122] Clinical trials evaluating the role of these agents in older patients with heart failure at discharge are needed.

Discharge planning is key, and follow-up should be individualized based on the patient's needs and capabilities. An outpatient follow-up visit for diabetes is generally recommended within 2 to 4 weeks of discharge if possible. Discharge recommendation should include medication reconciliation, structured communication with regard to medication changes, follow-up testing, and follow-up clinic appointment and contact information.[131] Home health referral can be used for those patients who are eligible, and if the referral lists diabetes as a concern in the consultation, glucose monitoring and diabetes care can be included. Patients under Medicare coverage are eligible if they are homebound and require skilled nursing care, physical/occupational therapy, or speech services.[132] If a patient requires full-time or extended skilled nursing care, home health is not applicable, and care would be taken over at the facility based on discharge recommendations.[132,133] In a recent RCT enrolling LTC residents (∼70 years), we observed that the use of a DPP-4 inhibitor can result in similar glycemic control along with a marked reduction in hypoglycemia when compared with low doses of basal insulin.[91]

SUMMARY

The number of adults living with diabetes has more than tripled during the past two decades, representing one of the fastest growing health challenges of the twenty-first century.[134] Patients with diabetes are more likely to be hospitalized compared with patients without diabetes. Among them, the most vulnerable are older patients with uncontrolled diabetes. In the hospital, more than half of all admitted patients with diabetes are older than 65 years; however, limited research has focused specifically on this population. Older patients with diabetes are commonly frail and have multiple comorbidities; therefore, an individualized patient-centered treatment approach is needed to avoid dangerous hypoglycemic and hyperglycemic events. Approaches with simplified regimens using agents with lower risk of hypoglycemia should be preferred for older patients with diabetes in the inpatient setting. Insulin therapy remains a useful drug for many elderly patients, such as those with moderate to severe hyperglycemia, history of hyperglycemic emergency, and those who fail to maintain glucose control with oral agents. Recent clinical trials have consistently shown that DPP-4 inhibitors alone or in combination with low doses of basal insulin have safety advantages and comparable efficacy to complex insulin therapy regimens.

DISCLOSURES

F.J. Pasquel has received consulting fees and research support from Merck and Dexcom, and consulting fees from Sanofi, Boehringer Ingelheim, Lilly, and AstraZeneca. G.E. Umpierrez has received unrestricted research support for inpatient studies (to Emory University) from Sanofi, Novo Nordisk, and Dexcom. A. Wallia has received research support from United Health Group, Eli Lilly, and Novo Nordisk. G.M. Davis and K. DeCarlo report no conflicts of interest.

REFERENCES

1. Cho NH, Shaw JE, Karuranga S, et al. IDF diabetes atlas: global estimates of diabetes prevalence for 2017 and projections for 2045. Diabetes Res Clin Pract 2018;138:271–81.
2. Bommer C, Sagalova V, Heesemann E, et al. Global economic burden of diabetes in adults: projections from 2015 to 2030. Diabetes Care 2018;41(5):963–70.
3. Bullard KM, Cowie CC, Lessem SE, et al. Prevalence of diagnosed diabetes in adults by diabetes type - United States, 2016. MMWR Morb Mortal Wkly Rep 2018;67(12):359–61.
4. Centers for Disease Control and Prevention. National hospital discharge survey "rate of discharges from short-stay hospitals, by age and first-listed diagnosis: United States, 2010". Available at: http://www.cdc.gov/nchs/data/nhds/3firstlisted/2010first3_rateage.pdf. Accessed July 2016.
5. Moghissi ES, Korytkowski MT, DiNardo M, et al. American Association of Clinical Endocrinologists and American Diabetes Association consensus statement on inpatient glycemic control. Diabetes Care 2009;32(6):1119–31.
6. McDonnell ME, Umpierrez GE. Insulin therapy for the management of hyperglycemia in hospitalized patients. Endocrinol Metab Clin North Am 2012;41(1):175–201.
7. Umpierrez GE, Smiley D, Jacobs S, et al. Randomized study of basal-bolus insulin therapy in the inpatient management of patients with type 2 diabetes undergoing general surgery (RABBIT 2 surgery). Diabetes Care 2011;34(2):256–61.
8. Investigators N-SS, Finfer S, Liu B, et al. Hypoglycemia and risk of death in critically ill patients. N Engl J Med 2012;367(12):1108–18.
9. Umpierrez GE, Pasquel FJ. Management of inpatient hyperglycemia and diabetes in older adults. Diabetes Care 2017;40(4):509–17.
10. Win TT, Davis HT, Laskey WK. Mortality among patients hospitalized with heart failure and diabetes mellitus: results from the national inpatient sample 2000 to 2010. Circ Heart Fail 2016;9(5):e003023.
11. American Diabetes A. Diagnosis and classification of diabetes mellitus. Diabetes Care 2009;32(Suppl 1):S62–7.
12. Diaz-Valencia PA, Bougneres P, Valleron AJ. Global epidemiology of type 1 diabetes in young adults and adults: a systematic review. BMC Public Health 2015;15:255.
13. Centers for Disease Control and Prevention. National diabetes statistics report, 2017. Atlanta (GA): Centers for Disease Control and Prevention, U.S. Dept of Health and Human Services; 2017.
14. Desai R, Singh S, Syed MH, et al. Temporal trends in the prevalence of diabetes decompensation (diabetic ketoacidosis and hyperosmolar hyperglycemic state) among adult patients hospitalized with diabetes mellitus: a nationwide analysis stratified by age, gender, and race. Cureus 2019;11(4):e4353.
15. American Diabetes Association. Economic costs of diabetes in the U.S. In 2017. Diabetes Care 2018;41(5):917–28.
16. Schmeltz LR, DeSantis AJ, Thiyagarajan V, et al. Reduction of surgical mortality and morbidity in diabetic patients undergoing cardiac surgery with a combined

intravenous and subcutaneous insulin glucose management strategy. Diabetes Care 2007;30(4):823–8.

17. van den Berghe G, Wouters P, Weekers F, et al. Intensive insulin therapy in the critically ill patients. N Engl J Med 2001;345(19):1359–67.

18. Umpierrez GE, Isaacs SD, Bazargan N, et al. Hyperglycemia: an independent marker of in-hospital mortality in patients with undiagnosed diabetes. J Clin Endocrinol Metab 2002;87(3):978–82.

19. Cook CB, Kongable GL, Potter DJ, et al. Inpatient glucose control: a glycemic survey of 126 U.S. hospitals. J Hosp Med 2009;4(9):E7–14.

20. Schneider AL, Kalyani RR, Golden S, et al. Diabetes and prediabetes and risk of hospitalization: the Atherosclerosis Risk in Communities (ARIC) study. Diabetes Care 2016;39(5):772–9.

21. Chia CW, Egan JM, Ferrucci L. Age-related changes in glucose metabolism, hyperglycemia, and cardiovascular risk. Circ Res 2018;123(7):886–904.

22. Lee PG, Halter JB. The pathophysiology of hyperglycemia in older adults: clinical considerations. Diabetes Care 2017;40(4):444–52.

23. Fink RI, Kolterman OG, Griffin J, et al. Mechanisms of insulin resistance in aging. J Clin Invest 1983;71(6):1523–35.

24. Defronzo RA. Glucose intolerance and aging: evidence for tissue insensitivity to insulin. Diabetes 1979;28(12):1095–101.

25. DeFronzo RA. Glucose intolerance and aging. Diabetes Care 1981;4(4):493–501.

26. Chen M, Bergman RN, Pacini G, et al. Pathogenesis of age-related glucose intolerance in man: insulin resistance and decreased beta-cell function. J Clin Endocrinol Metab 1985;60(1):13–20.

27. Szoke E, Shrayyef MZ, Messing S, et al. Effect of aging on glucose homeostasis: accelerated deterioration of beta-cell function in individuals with impaired glucose tolerance. Diabetes Care 2008;31(3):539–43.

28. Basu R, Breda E, Oberg AL, et al. Mechanisms of the age-associated deterioration in glucose tolerance: contribution of alterations in insulin secretion, action, and clearance. Diabetes 2003;52(7):1738–48.

29. Huang ES, Laiteerapong N, Liu JY, et al. Rates of complications and mortality in older patients with diabetes mellitus: the diabetes and aging study. JAMA Intern Med 2014;174(2):251–8.

30. Kirkman MS, Briscoe VJ, Clark N, et al. Diabetes in older adults: a consensus report. J Am Geriatr Soc 2012;60(12):2342–56.

31. Sinclair AJ, Abdelhafiz A, Dunning T, et al. An international position statement on the management of frailty in diabetes mellitus: summary of recommendations 2017. J Frailty Aging 2018;7(1):10–20.

32. Inouye SK, Studenski S, Tinetti ME, et al. Geriatric syndromes: clinical, research, and policy implications of a core geriatric concept. J Am Geriatr Soc 2007;55(5):780–91.

33. Araki A, Ito H. Diabetes mellitus and geriatric syndromes. Geriatr Gerontol Int 2009;9(2):105–14.

34. Jover N, Traissac T, Pinganaud G, et al. Varying insulin use in older hospitalized patients with diabetes. J Nutr Health Aging 2009;13(5):456–9.

35. Parker SG, McCue P, Phelps K, et al. What is Comprehensive Geriatric Assessment (CGA)? An umbrella review. Age and ageing 2018;47(1):149–55.

36. Medicare Learning Network Booklet. Annual wellness visit. In: Services USCf-MaM, U.S. Department of Health and Human Services (HHS). Baltimore (MD): American Medical Association; 2018:1–16. Available at: https://www.cms.gov/

Outreach-and-Education/Medicare-Learning-Network-MLN/MLNProducts/MLN-Publications-Items/CMS1246474. Accessed May 9, 2020.

37. LeRoith D, Biessels GJ, Braithwaite SS, et al. Treatment of diabetes in older adults: an Endocrine Society* clinical practice guideline. J Clin Endocrinol Metab 2019;104(5):1520–74.

38. Bourdel-Marchasson I, Sinclair A. Elderly patients with type 2 diabetes mellitus-the need for high-quality, inpatient diabetes care. Hosp Pract (1995) 2013; 41(4):51–6.

39. Pilotto A, Cella A, Pilotto A, et al. Three decades of comprehensive geriatric assessment: evidence coming from different healthcare settings and specific clinical conditions. J Am Med Dir Assoc 2017;18(2):192.e13-20.

40. Ellis G, Gardner M, Tsiachristas A, et al. Comprehensive geriatric assessment for older adults admitted to hospital. Cochrane Database Syst Rev 2017;(9):CD006211.

41. Older adults: standards of medical care in diabetes-2019. Diabetes Care 2019; 42(Suppl 1):S139–47.

42. Moreno G, Mangione CM, Kimbro L, et al. Guidelines abstracted from the American Geriatrics Society Guidelines for improving the care of older adults with diabetes mellitus: 2013 update. J Am Geriatr Soc 2013;61(11):2020–6.

43. Van Craen K, Braes T, Wellens N, et al. The effectiveness of inpatient geriatric evaluation and management units: a systematic review and meta-analysis. J Am Geriatr Soc 2010;58(1):83–92.

44. Halter J, Ouslander JG, Studenski S, et al. Hazzard's geriatric medicine and gerontology. 7th edition. New York: McGraw-Hill; 2017.

45. Aliberti MJR, Apolinario D, Suemoto CK, et al. Targeted geriatric assessment for fast-paced healthcare settings: development, validity, and reliability. J Am Geriatr Soc 2018;66(4):748–54.

46. Aliberti MJR, Covinsky KE, Apolinario D, et al. A 10-min targeted geriatric assessment predicts mortality in fast-paced acute care settings: a prospective cohort study. J Nutr Health Aging 2019;23(3):286–90.

47. Hopkins R, Shaver K, Weinstock RS. Management of adults with diabetes and cognitive problems. Diabetes Spectr 2016;29(4):224–37.

48. Borson S, Scanlan JM, Chen P, et al. The Mini-Cog as a screen for dementia: validation in a population-based sample. J Am Geriatr Soc 2003;51(10):1451–4.

49. Pasquier F. Diabetes and cognitive impairment: how to evaluate the cognitive status? Diabetes Metab 2010;36(Suppl 3):S100–5.

50. Woods NF, LaCroix AZ, Gray SL, et al. Frailty: emergence and consequences in women aged 65 and older in the Women's Health Initiative Observational Study. J Am Geriatr Soc 2005;53(8):1321–30.

51. Cawthon PM, Marshall LM, Michael Y, et al. Frailty in older men: prevalence, progression, and relationship with mortality. J Am Geriatr Soc 2007;55(8):1216–23.

52. Aguayo GA, Donneau AF, Vaillant MT, et al. Agreement between 35 published frailty scores in the general population. Am J Epidemiol 2017;186(4):420–34.

53. Apostolo J, Cooke R, Bobrowicz-Campos E, et al. Predicting risk and outcomes for frail older adults: an umbrella review of frailty screening tools. JBI Database Syst Rev Implement Rep 2017;15(4):1154–208.

54. Evans SJ, Sayers M, Mitnitski A, et al. The risk of adverse outcomes in hospitalized older patients in relation to a frailty index based on a comprehensive geriatric assessment. Age and ageing 2014;43(1):127–32.

55. MacKenzie HT, Tugwell B, Rockwood K, et al. Frailty and diabetes in older hospitalized adults: the case for routine frailty assessment. Can J Diabetes 2020; 44(3):241–5.e1.
56. Fox MT, Persaud M, Maimets I, et al. Effectiveness of acute geriatric unit care using acute care for elders components: a systematic review and meta-analysis. J Am Geriatr Soc 2012;60(12):2237–45.
57. Bansal V, Mottalib A, Pawar TK, et al. Inpatient diabetes management by specialized diabetes team versus primary service team in non-critical care units: impact on 30-day readmission rate and hospital cost. BMJ Open Diabetes Res Care 2018;6(1):e000460.
58. Mandel SR, Langan S, Mathioudakis NN, et al. Retrospective study of inpatient diabetes management service, length of stay and 30-day readmission rate of patients with diabetes at a community hospital. J Community Hosp Intern Med Perspect 2019;9(2):64–73.
59. Healy SJ, Black D, Harris C, et al. Inpatient diabetes education is associated with less frequent hospital readmission among patients with poor glycemic control. Diabetes Care 2013;36(10):2960–7.
60. Wexler DJ, Beauharnais CC, Regan S, et al. Impact of inpatient diabetes management, education, and improved discharge transition on glycemic control 12 months after discharge. Diabetes Res Clin Pract 2012;98(2):249–56.
61. Falciglia M, Freyberg RW, Almenoff PL, et al. Hyperglycemia-related mortality in critically ill patients varies with admission diagnosis. Crit Care Med 2009;37(12): 3001–9.
62. Siegelaar SE, Hermanides J, Oudemans-van Straaten HM, et al. Mean glucose during ICU admission is related to mortality by a U-shaped curve in surgical and medical patients: a retrospective cohort study. Crit Care 2010;14(6):R224.
63. Umpierrez GE, Hor T, Smiley D, et al. Comparison of inpatient insulin regimens with detemir plus aspart versus neutral protamine hagedorn plus regular in medical patients with type 2 diabetes. J Clin Endocrinol Metab 2009;94(2): 564–9.
64. Umpierrez GE, Smiley D, Zisman A, et al. Randomized study of basal-bolus insulin therapy in the inpatient management of patients with type 2 diabetes (RABBIT 2 trial). Diabetes Care 2007;30(9):2181–6.
65. Umpierrez GE, Smiley D, Hermayer K, et al. Randomized study comparing a basal-bolus with a basal plus correction insulin regimen for the hospital management of medical and surgical patients with type 2 diabetes: basal plus trial. Diabetes Care 2013;36(8):2169–74.
66. American Diabetes A. 15. Diabetes care in the hospital: standards of medical care in diabetes-2019. Diabetes Care 2019;42(Suppl 1):S173–81.
67. Lazar HL, McDonnell M, Chipkin SR, et al. The Society of Thoracic Surgeons practice guideline series: blood glucose management during adult cardiac surgery. Ann Thorac Surg 2009;87(2):663–9.
68. Lazar HL, McDonnell MM, Chipkin S, et al. Effects of aggressive versus moderate glycemic control on clinical outcomes in diabetic coronary artery bypass graft patients. Ann Surg 2011;254(3):458–63 [discussion: 463–4].
69. Umpierrez G, Cardona S, Pasquel F, et al. Randomized controlled trial of intensive versus conservative glucose control in patients undergoing coronary artery bypass graft surgery: GLUCO-CABG trial. Diabetes Care 2015;38(9):1665–72.
70. Pasquel FJ, Gomez-Huelgas R, Anzola I, et al. Predictive value of admission hemoglobin A1c on inpatient glycemic control and response to insulin therapy in

medicine and surgery patients with type 2 diabetes. Diabetes Care 2015;38(12): e202–3.

71. Umpierrez GE, Hellman R, Korytkowski MT, et al. Management of hyperglycemia in hospitalized patients in non-critical care setting: an endocrine society clinical practice guideline. J Clin Endocrinol Metab 2012;97(1):16–38.

72. Boucai L, Southern WN, Zonszein J. Hypoglycemia-associated mortality is not drug-associated but linked to comorbidities. Am J Med 2011;124(11):1028–35.

73. Vriesendorp TM, van Santen S, DeVries JH, et al. Predisposing factors for hypoglycemia in the intensive care unit. Crit Care Med 2006;34(1):96–101.

74. Farrokhi F, Klindukhova O, Chandra P, et al. Risk factors for inpatient hypoglycemia during subcutaneous insulin therapy in non-critically ill patients with type 2 diabetes. J Diabetes Sci Technol 2012;6(5):1022–9.

75. Kagansky N, Levy S, Rimon E, et al. Hypoglycemia as a predictor of mortality in hospitalized elderly patients. Arch Intern Med 2003;163(15):1825–9.

76. Stagnaro-Green A, Barton MK, Linekin PL, et al. Mortality in hospitalized patients with hypoglycemia and severe hyperglycemia. Mt Sinai J Med 1995;62(6): 422–6.

77. Shilo S, Berezovsky S, Friedlander Y, et al. Hypoglycemia in hospitalized nondiabetic older patients. J Am Geriatr Soc 1998;46(8):978–82.

78. Shorr RI, Ray WA, Daugherty JR, et al. Incidence and risk factors for serious hypoglycemia in older persons using insulin or sulfonylureas. Arch Intern Med 1997;157(15):1681–6.

79. Garg R, Hurwitz S, Turchin A, et al. Hypoglycemia, with or without insulin therapy, is associated with increased mortality among hospitalized patients. Diabetes Care 2013;36(5):1107–10.

80. Kosiborod M, Inzucchi SE, Goyal A, et al. Relationship between spontaneous and iatrogenic hypoglycemia and mortality in patients hospitalized with acute myocardial infarction. JAMA 2009;301(15):1556–64.

81. Wexler DJ, Meigs JB, Cagliero E, et al. Prevalence of hyper- and hypoglycemia among inpatients with diabetes: a national survey of 44 U.S. hospitals. Diabetes Care 2007;30(2):367–9.

82. Newton CA, Adeel A, Sadeghi-Yarandi S, et al. Prevalence, quality of care and complications in long-term care residents with diabetes: a multicenter observational study. J Am Med Dir Assoc 2013;14(11):842–6.

83. Bueno E, Benitez A, Rufinelli JV, et al. Basal-bolus regimen with insulin analogues versus human insulin in medical patients with type 2 diabetes: a randomized controlled trial in Latin America. Endocr Pract 2015;21(7):807–13.

84. Wilson M, Weinreb J, Hoo GW. Intensive insulin therapy in critical care: a review of 12 protocols. Diabetes Care 2007;30(4):1005–11.

85. Jacobi J, Bircher N, Krinsley J, et al. Guidelines for the use of an insulin infusion for the management of hyperglycemia in critically ill patients. Crit Care Med 2012;40(12):3251–76.

86. Bellido V, Suarez L, Rodriguez MG, et al. Comparison of basal-bolus and premixed insulin regimens in hospitalized patients with type 2 diabetes. Diabetes Care 2015;38(12):2211–6.

87. Franchin A, Maran A, Bruttomesso D, et al. The GesTIO protocol experience: safety of a standardized order set for subcutaneous insulin regimen in elderly hospitalized patients. Aging Clin Exp Res 2017;29(6):1087–93.

88. Pasquel FJ, Fayfman M, Umpierrez GE. Debate on insulin vs non-insulin use in the hospital setting-is it time to revise the guidelines for the management of inpatient diabetes? Curr Diab Rep 2019;19(9):65.

89. Pasquel FJ, Powell W, Peng L, et al. A randomized controlled trial comparing treatment with oral agents and basal insulin in elderly patients with type 2 diabetes in long-term care facilities. BMJ open Diabetes Res Care 2015;3(1): e000104.

90. Umpierrez GE, Korytkowski M. Is incretin-based therapy ready for the care of hospitalized patients with type 2 diabetes? Insulin therapy has proven itself and is considered the mainstay of treatment. Diabetes Care 2013;36(7):2112–7.

91. Umpierrez GE, Cardona S, Chachkhiani D, et al. A randomized controlled study comparing a DPP4 inhibitor (Linagliptin) and basal insulin (Glargine) in patients with type 2 diabetes in long-term care and skilled nursing facilities: linagliptin-LTC trial. J Am Med Dir Assoc 2018;19(5):399–404.e3.

92. Schwartz SS, DeFronzo RA, Umpierrez GE. Practical implementation of incretin-based therapy in hospitalized patients with type 2 diabetes. Postgrad Med 2015;127(2):251–7.

93. Jespersen MJ, Knop FK, Christensen M. GLP-1 agonists for type 2 diabetes: pharmacokinetic and toxicological considerations. Expert Opin Drug Metab Toxicol 2013;9(1):17–29.

94. Marso SP, Bain SC, Consoli A, et al. Semaglutide and cardiovascular outcomes in patients with type 2 diabetes. N Engl J Med 2016;375(19):1834–44.

95. Marso SP, Daniels GH, Brown-Frandsen K, et al. Liraglutide and cardiovascular outcomes in type 2 diabetes. N Engl J Med 2016;375(4):311–22.

96. Holman RR, Bethel MA, Mentz RJ, et al. Effects of once-weekly exenatide on cardiovascular outcomes in type 2 diabetes. N Engl J Med 2017;377(13): 1228–39.

97. Hernandez AF, Green JB, Janmohamed S, et al. Albiglutide and cardiovascular outcomes in patients with type 2 diabetes and cardiovascular disease (Harmony Outcomes): a double-blind, randomised placebo-controlled trial. Lancet 2018; 392(10157):1519–29.

98. Pasquel FJ, Gianchandani R, Rubin DJ, et al. Efficacy of sitagliptin for the hospital management of general medicine and surgery patients with type 2 diabetes (Sita-Hospital): a multicentre, prospective, open-label, non-inferiority randomised trial. Lancet Diabetes Endocrinol 2017;5(2):125–33.

99. Umpierrez GE, Gianchandani R, Smiley D, et al. Safety and efficacy of sitagliptin therapy for the inpatient management of general medicine and surgery patients with type 2 diabetes: a pilot, randomized, controlled study. Diabetes Care 2013; 36(11):3430–5.

100. Vellanki P, Rasouli N, Baldwin D, et al. Glycaemic efficacy and safety of linagliptin compared to basal-bolus insulin regimen in patients with type 2 diabetes undergoing non-cardiac surgery: a multicenter randomized clinical trial. Diabetes Obes Metab 2019;21(4):837–43.

101. Garg R, Schuman B, Hurwitz S, et al. Safety and efficacy of saxagliptin for glycemic control in non-critically ill hospitalized patients. BMJ open Diabetes Res Care 2017;5(1):e000394.

102. Perez-Belmonte LM, Gomez-Doblas JJ, Millan-Gomez M, et al. Use of linagliptin for the management of medicine department inpatients with type 2 diabetes in real-world clinical practice (Lina-Real-World Study). J Clin Med 2018;7(9) [pii: E271].

103. Nystrom T, Gutniak MK, Zhang Q, et al. Effects of glucagon-like peptide-1 on endothelial function in type 2 diabetes patients with stable coronary artery disease. Am J Physiol Endocrinol Metab 2004;287(6):E1209–15.

104. Lonborg J, Kelbaek H, Vejlstrup N, et al. Exenatide reduces final infarct size in patients with ST-segment-elevation myocardial infarction and short-duration of ischemia. Circ Cardiovasc Interv 2012;5(2):288–95.

105. Sokos GG, Nikolaidis LA, Mankad S, et al. Glucagon-like peptide-1 infusion improves left ventricular ejection fraction and functional status in patients with chronic heart failure. J Card Fail 2006;12(9):694–9.

106. Nathanson D, Ullman B, Lofstrom U, et al. Effects of intravenous exenatide in type 2 diabetic patients with congestive heart failure: a double-blind, randomised controlled clinical trial of efficacy and safety. Diabetologia 2012;55(4): 926–35.

107. Sokos GG, Bolukoglu H, German J, et al. Effect of glucagon-like peptide-1 (GLP-1) on glycemic control and left ventricular function in patients undergoing coronary artery bypass grafting. Am J Cardiol 2007;100(5):824–9.

108. Nikolaidis LA, Mankad S, Sokos GG, et al. Effects of glucagon-like peptide-1 in patients with acute myocardial infarction and left ventricular dysfunction after successful reperfusion. Circulation 2004;109(8):962–5.

109. Abuannadi M, Kosiborod M, Riggs L, et al. Management of hyperglycemia with the administration of intravenous exenatide to patients in the cardiac intensive care unit. Endocr Pract 2013;19(1):81–90.

110. Besch G, Perrotti A, Mauny F, et al. Clinical effectiveness of intravenous exenatide infusion in perioperative glycemic control after coronary artery bypass graft surgery: a phase II/III randomized trial. Anesthesiology 2017;127(5):775–87.

111. Polderman JAW, van Steen SCJ, Thiel B, et al. Peri-operative management of patients with type-2 diabetes mellitus undergoing non-cardiac surgery using liraglutide, glucose-insulin-potassium infusion or intravenous insulin bolus regimens: a randomised controlled trial. Anaesthesia 2018;73(3):332–9.

112. Kohl BA, Hammond MS, Cucchiara AJ, et al. Intravenous GLP-1 (7-36) amide for prevention of hyperglycemia during cardiac surgery: a randomized, double-blind, placebo-controlled study. J Cardiothorac Vasc Anesth 2014;28(3): 618–25.

113. Besch G, Perrotti A, Salomon du Mont L, et al. Impact of intravenous exenatide infusion for perioperative blood glucose control on myocardial ischemia-reperfusion injuries after coronary artery bypass graft surgery: sub study of the phase II/III ExSTRESS randomized trial. Cardiovasc Diabetol 2018; 17(1):140.

114. Hulst AH, Visscher MJ, Godfried MB, et al. Study protocol of the randomised placebo-controlled GLOBE trial: GLP-1 for bridging of hyperglycaemia during cardiac surgery. BMJ open 2018;8(6):e022189.

115. Hulst AH, Preckel B, Hollman MW, et al. Liraglutide for perioperative management of hyperglycaemia in cardiac surgery patients (GLOBE): a multicentre, prospective, superiority randomised trial. In. Vol Diabetes 2019 June; 68(Supplement 1). 79th Annual Meeting of the American Diabetes Association: American Diabetes Association; 2019.

116. Fayfman M, Galindo RJ, Rubin DJ, et al. A randomized controlled trial on the safety and efficacy of exenatide therapy for the inpatient management of general medicine and surgery patients with type 2 diabetes. Diabetes Care 2019; 42(3):450–6.

117. Fayfman M, Anzola I, Urrutia MA, et al. 1007-P: incretin therapy with DPP-4-I and GLP1-RA for the hospital management of elderly adults with type 2 diabetes. Diabetes 2019;68(Supplement 1):1007.

118. Hsia DS, Grove O, Cefalu WT. An update on sodium-glucose co-transporter-2 inhibitors for the treatment of diabetes mellitus. Curr Opin Endocrinol Diabetes Obes 2017;24(1):73–9.
119. Zinman B, Wanner C, Lachin JM, et al. Empagliflozin, cardiovascular outcomes, and mortality in type 2 diabetes. N Engl J Med 2015;373(22):2117–28.
120. Neal B, Perkovic V, Mahaffey KW, et al. Canagliflozin and cardiovascular and renal events in type 2 diabetes. N Engl J Med 2017;377(7):644–57.
121. Perkovic V, Jardine MJ, Neal B, et al. Canagliflozin and renal outcomes in type 2 diabetes and nephropathy. N Engl J Med 2019;380(24):2295–306.
122. Monteiro P, Bergenstal RM, Toural E, et al. Efficacy and safety of empagliflozin in older patients in the EMPA-REG OUTCOME(R) trial. Age and ageing 2019;48(6): 859–66.
123. Singh LG, Levitt DL, Satyarengga M, et al. Continuous glucose monitoring in general wards for prevention of hypoglycemia: results from the glucose telemetry system pilot study. J Diabetes Sci Technol 2019. 1932296819889640. [epub ahead of print].
124. Bally L, Thabit H, Hartnell S, et al. Closed-loop insulin delivery for glycemic control in noncritical care. N Engl J Med 2018;379(6):547–56.
125. Blaum C, Cigolle CT, Boyd C, et al. Clinical complexity in middle-aged and older adults with diabetes: the Health and Retirement Study. Med Care 2010;48(4): 327–34.
126. Umpierrez GE, Reyes D, Smiley D, et al. Hospital discharge algorithm based on admission HbA1c for the management of patients with type 2 diabetes. Diabetes Care 2014;37(11):2934–9.
127. Munshi MN, Slyne C, Segal AR, et al. Simplification of insulin regimen in older adults and risk of hypoglycemia. JAMA Intern Med 2016;176(7):1023–5.
128. Shankar RR, Xu L, Golm GT, et al. A comparison of glycaemic effects of sitagliptin and sulfonylureas in elderly patients with type 2 diabetes mellitus. Int J Clin Pract 2015;69(6):626–31.
129. Ledesma G, Umpierrez GE, Morley JE, et al. Efficacy and safety of linagliptin to improve glucose control in older people with type 2 diabetes on stable insulin therapy: a randomized trial. Diabetes Obes Metab 2019;21(11):2465–73.
130. Gianchandani RY, Pasquel FJ, Rubin DJ, et al. The efficacy and safety of co-administration of sitagliptin with metformin in patients with type 2 diabetes at hospital discharge. Endocr Pract 2018;24(6):556–64.
131. Diabetes care in the hospital: standards of medical care in diabetes-2018. Diabetes Care 2018;41(Suppl 1):S144–51.
132. Centers for Medicare and Medicaid Services. Medicare and Home Health Care. In: Services USDoHaH, U.S. Department of Health and Human Services. Baltimore (MD): 2017. Vol. 10969. 1–32. Available at: https://www.medicare.gov/Pubs/pdf/10969-Medicare-and-Home-Health-Care.pdf. Accessed May 9, 2020.
133. Linekin PL. Home health care and diabetes assesment, care, and education, vol. 16. Diabetes Spectrum: a Publication of the American Diabetes Association; 2003. p. 217–22, 4.
134. International Diabetes Federation. IDF diabetes atlas. 9th edition 2019. Brussels (Belgium): Available at: http://www.diabetesatlas.org. Accessed May 9, 2020.

Artificial Intelligence and Digital Tools
Future of Diabetes Care

Ram D. Sriram, PhD[a],*, S. Sethu K. Reddy, MD, MBA[b]

KEYWORDS

- Artificial intelligence • Diabetes mellitus • Natural language processing
- Knowledge-based expert systems • Neural networks • P7 medicine

KEY POINTS

- The symbiosis of Internet of things and social networks—called the Internet of everything—will have significant implications on health care delivery.
- Advances in computer hardware facilitated multilayered neural networks, which led to significant improvements in machine learning.
- Artificial intelligence can be applied to various types of problems that arise in diabetes care: clinical diagnosis, interpretation, monitoring, developing treatment plans, and designing drugs.
- Artificial intelligence may be able to translate clinical practice guidelines to implementable decision support systems.

INTRODUCTION

Artificial intelligence (AI) can be defined as a means for computers to do tasks that would normally require human intelligence.[1] Diabetes mellitus is a chronic, pervasive condition that is data rich and with a variety of potential outcomes. Thus, diabetes is fertile ground for incorporating AI.[2] Sample questions clinicians often pose include: How will this individual respond to a specific medication? Who will develop diabetic retinopathy? How can we generate a personalized glucose control algorithm to help develop a safe closed loop system? Which of my patients are at risk of influenza this fall? Of the millions with prediabetes, who is most likely to develop diabetes and thus benefit from preventive regimens?

At this time, most individuals have become part of a vibrant, changing ecosystem, where one's social, biologic and other variables are accessible to interested parties.

[a] National Institute of Standards and Technology, 100 Bureau Drive, MS 8970, National Institute of Standards and Technology, Gaithersburg, MD 20899, USA; [b] Department of Internal, CMED 2419, Central Michigan University, Mt. Pleasant, MI 48859, USA
* Corresponding author.
E-mail address: sriram@nist.gov

Clin Geriatr Med 36 (2020) 513–525
https://doi.org/10.1016/j.cger.2020.04.009
0749-0690/20/© 2020 Elsevier Inc. All rights reserved.

geriatric.theclinics.com

Although privacy regulations about the access to this data by third parties will no doubt be put in place, once an individual permits sharing his or her data, AI will lead to more confident recommendations for that individual. With advances in machine learning and deep learning along with improved natural language processing, AI should lead to more timely, validated advice.

The journey to future health care will involve advances in mainly 3 dimensions: (1) advances in health care technology, (2) advances in health care delivery, and (3) advances in computer science and information technology. Advances in health care technology include breakthroughs in the human genome project, pharmaceuticals and nutraceuticals, and medical devices.[3] In health care practice, we have novel methods developed for better disease management, evidence-based health care across the continuum of care, and mind–body medicine.[4] Innovations in computer science and information technology are helping to handle and understand the vast amount of health information (we will use the abbreviation IT to denote computer science and information technology). These innovations are happening in speed and storage capacity, mobile personal computing and communication devices, cloud computing, AI, networking, and biometrics. The Internet, which has spanned several networks in a wide variety of domains, is having a significant impact on every aspect of our lives. The next generation of networks will use a wide variety of resources with significant sensing and intelligent capabilities. Such networks will extend beyond physically linked computers to include multimodal information from biological, cognitive, semantic, and social networks. This paradigm shift will involve symbiotic networks of intelligent medical devices (implantable, injectable, on-body), and smart phones or mobile personal computing and communication devices. These devices—and the network—will be constantly sensing, monitoring, and interpreting the environment; this is sometimes referred to as the *Internet of things*. The symbiosis of the Internet of things and social networks—called the Internet of everything—will have significant implications on the way health care is delivered in the United States.

The P4 medicine concept[5] pioneered by Leroy Hood, Institute of Systems Biology, has been extended to the P7 concept (personal communication—Sriram and Jain, 2017). Elements of the P7 concept of the future of health care include the following elements.

1. *Personalized.* Personalized medicine involves tailoring/customizing treatment to each individual.
2. *Predictive.* Based on the information in the electronic health records and genomic data, we should be able to determine an individual's susceptibility to particular diseases.
3. *Precise.* Once data and information are gathered, then decision analytical tools can be used to precisely determine the cause of a disease and to recommend appropriate therapeutic actions.
4. *Preventive.* Instead of treating a disease when it inflicts a person, machine learning and decision analytical tools can be used to develop strategies to prevent the onset of disease.
5. *Pervasive.* The health care should be provided anytime, anywhere, and at any location.
6. *Participatory.* The patient should actively participate in the diagnosis and the treatment of his or her medical condition.
7. *Protective.* Appropriate safety measures should be taken to ensure that the confidentiality of all patient data is maintained.

All of these concepts will draw on the advances in AI, which are reviewed herein.

ARTIFICIAL INTELLIGENCE

Since the 1950s, when AI was conceived, AI has been deeply concerned with the understanding of human problem-solving strategies and incorporating (or simulating) these strategies into computer programs. The 1980s were dominated with the rise of knowledge-based systems, called the first wave. The second wave in the 2000s included advances in computer hardware–facilitated multilayered neural networks, which led to significant improvements in machine learning for certain classes of problems. Now, we are witnessing the third wave, which includes a combination of neural networks and knowledge structures.[6]

A general architecture of an intelligent agent is shown in **Fig. 1**. Perception forms the input to the intelligent agent in the form of vision, speech, touch, smell, and taste. Based on the input, the intelligent agent, using its reasoning apparatus, will take an appropriate action, which may involve language and/or manipulation. The reasoning apparatus will use knowledge and problem-solving techniques to process the input. In a machine environment we generally have automated natural language and speech processing programs for both input and output. The reasoning apparatus will contain knowledge in an appropriate representation scheme, general inference mechanisms, and machine learning techniques.[7]

From Data to Knowledge

It is a popular belief that data are abundant, but knowledge is scarce. Data are the raw form of signals that is generally transformed into information. Data are generally available in the form of observations, computational results, and factual quantities. Interpretation, abstraction, or association of the data leads to generation of information. Importantly, knowledge is obtained by experiencing and learning from this information and putting it into action. Knowledge can be represented in several ways. Common schemes are rules (IF–THEN), logic, objects and associated networks (eg, IF the HbA1c is >6.5%, THEN the individual is deemed to have the diagnosis of diabetes). As a further example, consider funduscopic images that consisting of megabytes of pixels, which can be abstracted into features (information). Using these features one can infer, using strategies described elsewhere in this article, if a person has diabetic retinopathy.

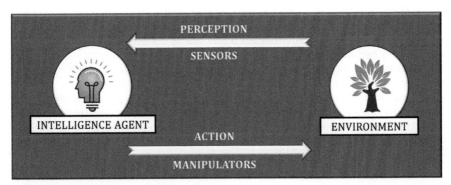

Fig. 1. Architecture of an intelligent agent.

Inference Mechanisms or Problem-Solving Techniques

When data or information stream into an intelligent agent, it is generally stored in a place called context, which is also known as short-term working memory. This data or information is acted on by several problem-solving techniques (also known as inference mechanisms).[8]

Knowledge-Based Expert Systems

Knowledge-based expert systems offer a convenient way to encode human knowledge and perform reasoning. These systems were very popular in the 1980s and several medical applications were developed (eg, MYCIN, INTERNIST). Later commercial systems, such as ILLIAD, were marketed.[9] There is always a need to know why certain decisions have been made (eg, Why did I get diabetes? Why did I develop renal disease? Why did I get shingles? Why did the computer say this cell was cancerous? What is the likelihood of catching the flu?). MYCIN was initially developed as a diagnostic tool for infectious diseases, and a module was incorporated to provide such explanations, both why certain questions were asked and also why certain decision paths were not taken. A domain independent version of MYCIN—called EMYCIN—was developed and this provided a framework for the development of knowledge-based expert systems in several domains[10] (eg, SACON in structural engineering). EMYCIN retained the explanation module incorporated in the original MYCIN framework. Several other domain independent tools were developed in the late 1980s and early 1990s.

Machine Learning

When new concepts and knowledge structures are generated by a computer, we call it machine learning.[11] There are essentially 3 components to machine learning: (1) data, (2) features, and (3) algorithms. Once extracted from the data, algorithms are applied to these features to learn new concepts or rules. Based on the amount of control over the output, machine learning can be categorized into supervised, unsupervised (or self-supervised), or reinforcement learning.[12] In supervised learning,[13] the system is given volumes of input data and the goal is to predict the output based on the input. In supervised learning, models are built or learned from labeled training data—an external agent, normally human, provides the correct (or ground-truth) label during training from which a model is learned. For example, input could be a large amount of glucose monitoring data and a patient's activity and food intake data and the output could be decision on prediction of hypoglycemia. In unsupervised learning, the machine learning algorithm may take the data and generate patterns without any external input. For example, the same data may be analyzed to lead to a de novo association or output. Machine learning may lead to identification of clusters of subjects that respond to various foods quite differently. Finally, in reinforcement learning (also known as semisupervised learning), the intelligent agent learns concepts through reward and failure, using certain optimization techniques. For example, reinforcement learning has been used in robotics to enable a robot to discover an optimal path through trial and error interactions with its environment.[14] Over the last few decades, machine learning algorithms rooted in statistics or logic-based reasoning have been developed. One such technique—called neural networks—that has gained considerable traction in medical AI applications in the recent past, is discussed elsewhere in this article.

Neural Networks

A neural network is a highly interconnected network of many simple processors or neurons and attempts to simulate the neuronal connections in the brain. Each neuron

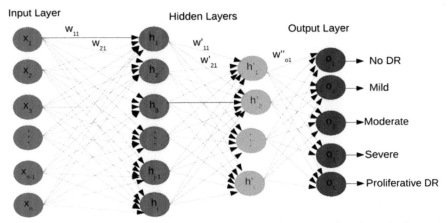

Fig. 2. Sample neural network. DR, diabetic retinopathy. (*Courtesy of* Sarala Padi, PhD, Gaithersburg, Maryland.)

in the network maintains only 1 piece of dynamic information (its current level of activation) and is capable of only a few simple computations (adding inputs, computing a new activation level, or comparing input to a threshold value). As shown in **Fig. 2**, a neural network model consists of input, output, and 1 or more hidden layers.[15] The number of neurons in the input and the output layers of the model is fixed depending on the given input size and the expected output size. For instance, if we are modeling the eye retina images for detecting diabetic retinopathy severity then the input layer size is fixed to image size (assuming input image size is $256 \times 256 = 65,536$ pixels) and the output size is fixed to 5, assuming that we are predicting 5 stages of diabetic retinopathy for the given input image. In contrast, the number of hidden layers and the number of neurons used in each hidden layer are not fixed. These are chosen empirically depending on the given problem.

Each neuron is weighted according to its connections with other neurons. The connection from an input neuron to an output neuron is simply a summation of neuron weights. However, the activation function applied on the summation learns the nonlinear relationship between the input and the output. Although neural network models were used to solve complex problems, these models were computationally expensive. Specifically for image processing applications, the input size and complexity increases with increasing image size.

To overcome these issues, convolutional neural network models were introduced, and these models have shown tremendous success in computational vision tasks. As shown in **Fig. 2**, a convolutional neural network model consists of convolutional and hidden layers that are connected to each other.[16] Convolutional layers extract features automatically from the given input image, and the hidden layers learn the nonlinear relationship between the given input and the output. The main advantage of the convolutional neural network model is that it does automatic feature engineering and convolutional layers share the parameters. The relationship between AI, ML, KBES, and NNs is shown in **Fig. 3**.

Kinds of Problems that Artificial Intelligence Is Being Used for

AI can be applied to various types of problems that arise in diabetes care. These problems can range from clinical diagnosis, interpretation, monitoring, developing treatment plans, and designing drugs.

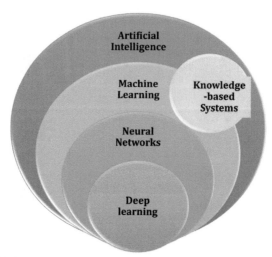

Fig. 3. Relationship between AI, machine learning, and neural networks (Overlap with KBS shown because some KBS have machine learning incorporated in them).

Diagnosis
The problems or diseases are identified based on potentially noisy data. The diagnostician must be able to relate the symptoms to the appropriate disease(s). The task may involve reasoning with incomplete and inexact data, faulty sensors, and so on. Diagnosis is usually followed by a treatment plan, where a set of actions to cure or treat the disease is determined.

Interpretation
The given data are analyzed to determine their meaning. The data are often either unreliable, erroneous, or extraneous. Hence, the system should be able to eliminate candidates based on incomplete information.

Monitoring
Signals are continuously interpreted and alarms are set whenever required.

Control
Signals or data are interpreted, and the system is regulated, based on deviations from expected response.

Treatment planning
A program of actions is set up to achieve certain goals. The course of actions should be set up such that excessive resources are not expended and/or constraints are not violated.

Drug design
Drugs that satisfy particular requirements can be configured. This type of problem involves satisfying constraints from a variety of sources. Large design problems are usually solved by dividing the problems into a number of subtasks. The designer must be able to handle the interactions between these subtasks properly.

AREAS OF ARTIFICIAL INTELLIGENCE USE IN DIABETES

In this section, we discuss several examples, where AI techniques are being applied in the treatment and management of diabetes.

Evolution to Closed-Loop System: Continuous Glucose Monitoring and Insulin Therapy

One major issue in managing diabetes is leveraging continuous glucose monitoring (CGM) data and insulin therapeutic decisions. There are several commercially available CGM devices.[17] CGM devices[18] have 3 primary components: (1) sensors (could be minimally invasive or noninvasive); (2) a transmitter, which transmits sensor readings; and (3) a receiver, which receives the sensor data and has software that can analyze the data. Nowadays, smart phones (iPhone, Android phone) act as receivers—either through a cloud or a Bluetooth interface. Software on a smart phone interprets the incoming sensor data, along with other data from a personal health record (**Figs. 4** and **5**), and detects various patterns. Based on an appropriate inference technique (and earlier rules learned through machine learning techniques), the insulin monitor will receive commands to make adjustments to the amount of insulin being pumped. For example, IBM Watson, in collaboration with Medtronic[19] developed an AI-based app called Sugar.IQ. There are other systems that can take images or get data from the web and can also determine the kinds of foods that you can eat.[20] Using all these data and various knowledge bases can aid in ensuring that the right types of food are eaten and diabetes is appropriately controlled.

A patient with diabetes must often calculate insulin dosage based on current blood sugar, previous blood sugar trends, nature of caloric intake, activity level, and other variables. This is a perfect scenario for incorporating AI. Recently, case-based reasoning has been incorporated into a bolus calculator, which is superior to existing calculators.[21] Such tools can be conveniently placed on a smartphone platform.

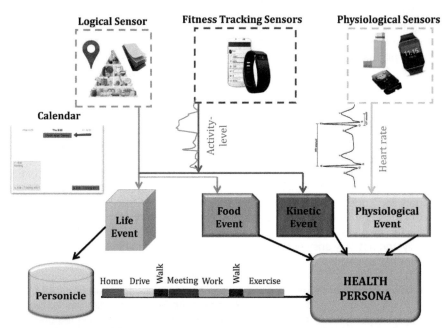

Fig. 4. Defining a health persona. (*Courtesy of* Dr. Ramesh Jain, PhD, Irvine, CA.)

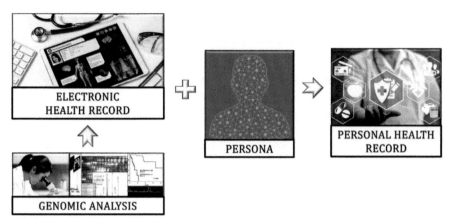

Fig. 5. A personal health record.

The Juvenile Diabetes Research Foundation launched the Artificial Pancreas Project in 2006 to develop a commercially available closed-loop system, using continuous subcutaneous insulin infusion linked with CGM to duplicate physiologic response to changes in glucose.[22] Fuzzy logic may help in refining these algorithms be more practical in real-life settings.[23] Early proof-of-concept studies of automated closed-loop insulin delivery systems have suggested that we are inching closer to an artificial pancreas.[24]

Analyzing Images that Can Give Clues to Diabetes (Google Retinopathy Detection)

Individuals with diabetes may experience a plethora of eye complications, including age-related macular degeneration, cataracts, glaucoma, and diabetic retinopathy. Among these disease, age-related macular degeneration affects 10 million people, who are over 50 years of age, in the United States. Diabetic retinopathy is a leading cause of blindness globally. Early diagnosis and management is key to preventing blindness. Because there are millions of individuals with diabetes eligible for early screening and necessary interventions, there is limited access to ophthalmology expertise. Hence, there is a considerable demand for an automated, high-sensitivity system for diabetic retinopathy detection. The automated methods can provide many benefits such as increasing the efficiency, reproducible results, coverage of screening programs, decreasing barriers to access, and improving patient outcomes by providing early detection.

AI can play a role not only in the diagnosis of diabetic retinopathy, but also in the severity of retinopathy. A further role of AI would be in analysis of the data to answer unsupervised questions. Traditional machine learning techniques can review extracted features and make the diagnosis and the severity of that diagnosis. Deep learning techniques—based on layers of neural networks—can extract features automatically and not only answer the original question of retinopathy diagnosis, but also show correlations with apparently unrelated outcomes.

This deep learning model optimizes the parameters using a mechanism called backpropagation, such that model parameters can be fine tuned to desired output of the model. For instance, **Fig. 6**) shows an example deep learning model architecture for diabetic retinopathy severity detection.[25] Initial layers extract low-level features and the final layers learn the high-level features for diabetic retinopathy diagnosis analysis.

Considerable work has been done on the automatic detection of diabetic retinopathy severity using deep learning models.[26] The deep learning model outperformed traditional machine learning models without explicitly extracting the features, identifying diabetic retinopathy in retinal fundus images with high sensitivity and specificity. The deep learning model, which can automatically diagnose diabetic retinopathy from the given images, has several advantages. These advantages include no need for manual pixel-level annotations, consistency, interpretation, high sensitivity, specificity,[27] and speed[28] in analyzing the images.[29]

Although deep learning models were successful in detecting the severity of diabetic retinopathy just by processing the images, these models have certain limitations. The main limitations are the need for large amounts of true diabetic retinopathy data,[30] the presence of significantly more prevalent nondiabetic retinopathy data, and the need for annotated data.[28] Because it is expensive to generate huge volumes of data for training the deep learning models, there is a need to design deep learning models that can learn from limited data.[31] One possibility can be exploration of generative adversarial networks models to automatically generate new samples from the given images.

Using Natural Language Processing to Scan Texts for Diabetes-Related Information

Semantic-driven medical information systems of the future will provide intelligent interfaces for medical researchers, doctors, and patients involving the use of medical information sources and intelligent medical devices. These intelligent interfaces will support information search, navigation, and modeling based on automated query expansion and the construction and use of information structures, such as term and document clustering, taxonomies, and ontologies of multiple very large corpora. The interfaces for the different stakeholder perspectives to the semantic representations will enable search, analysis, discovery, and communication across expert/nonexpert understanding and practice boundaries. They will need to support the constant sensing, monitoring, and interpreting of multimodal information from biological, cognitive, semantic, and social networks. The underlying infrastructure for these interfaces will have to be built and kept up to date. The critical problem is to embed this infrastructure in the practice of medicine.

The technology for this infrastructure requires composition of several AI technologies for neurolinguistic programming including a technology that was developed by the National Institute of Science and Technology: the root and rule-based analysis.[32]

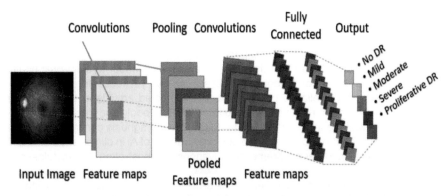

Fig. 6. A convolutional neural network model to detect diabetic retinopathy from the images. (*Courtesy of* Sarala Padi, PhD, Gaithersburg, Maryland.)

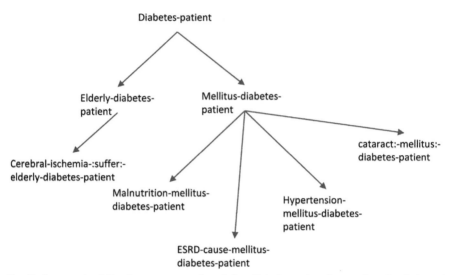

Fig. 7. Fragment of the taxonomy produced for diabetes using the root and rule-based method. ESRD, end-stage renal disease. (*Courtesy of* Eswaran Subrahmanian, PhD, Gaithersburg, Maryland.)

The National Institute of Science and Technology system combines neural networks, phrase-based parsing, and other neurolinguistic programming tools including latent semantic indexing. These strategies enable automated terminology and taxonomy extraction from very large medical documents that can improve searches on web sites such as PubMed. This approach provides automated query expansion using the derived taxonomic structures, such as shown in **Fig. 7**. Further, the National Institute of Science and Technology technique can be used to create topic-based document clusters. For example, documents that have terms relating to eye disease and diabetes can be filed in a single folder.

Clinical practice guidelines are constantly being updated with the latest evidence but are often bulky and burdensome to incorporate into one's practice. Using rule-based reasoning, it may be possible to translate guidelines to implementable decision support systems.[33] Recent experience with such a decision support system demonstrated that an improvement in self-monitoring can occur in the management of gestational diabetes.[34]

SUMMARY

The first AI systems were knowledge-based decision support systems, using stand-alone static datasets. Once these systems were able to connect to electronic health data, AI became useful for teaching purposes, but not yet ready for clinical care. Deep learning through reliance on multilayered connected artificial neural networks has led to potential clinical utility. In May 2019, teams at Google and New York University reported that deep learning models for lung cancer diagnosis can improve accuracy.[35] Although it is easy to exaggerate our expectations of AI in clinical medicine and in diabetes, there have been incremental advances demonstrating the usefulness of AI.

AI can be helpful in the development of the artificial pancreas (closed-loop systems) and in understanding the interplay between social determinants and physiologic biomarkers of health. Diabetes also generates a tremendous volume of retinal, renal, vascular, and other data, which can be tracked over time. Overlaying these patho-physiologic data with other seemingly unrelated data will no doubt lead to new insights into diabetes control and complications. The refinement of these processes will increase access to expert opinions and expert care to patients from all over the globe. A woman with diabetes in rural Africa will potentially be able to access eye care thousands of miles away via the use of her personal smart phone images. Instead of 1 algorithmic solution for all, glucose control algorithms can be personalized for the individual patient based on glucose excursions, insulin pharmacology, nutrigenomics, and activity/exercise patterns.

It is clear that we are on the cusp of a revolution in health care, with the ability to collect, analyze, and harness the wealth of data to lead to sage clinical advice. AI will play a significant role in transforming health care. We will also need further progress in knowledge representation and reasoning.[36]

DISCLAIMER AND ACKNOWLEDGMENTS

Certain commercial systems are identified in this article. Such identification does not imply recommendation or endorsement by NIST; nor does it imply that the products identified are necessarily the best available for the purpose. Further, any opinions, findings, conclusions or recommendations expressed in this material are those of the authors and do not necessarily reflect the views of NIST, other supporting U.S. government or corporate organizations. The authors would like to thank the following people for input into this document: Eswaran Subrahmanian, Sarala Padi, T.N. Bhat, Ramesh Jain, Kristina Rigopoulos (for the figures), Elham Tabassi, and NIST's internal review board.

DISCLOSURE

The authors have nothing to disclose.

REFERENCES

1. Boden M. Educational implications of artificial intelligence. In: Maxwell W, editor. Thinking: the expanding frontier. Proceedings of the International Conference on Thinking, University of the South Pacific, January, 1982. Philadelphia: The Franklin Institute Press, 1983. P. 227–31.

2. Rigla M, García-Sáez G, Pons B, et al. Artificial intelligence methodologies and their application to diabetes. J Diabetes Sci Technol 2018;12(2):303–10.

3. Hollis KF, Soualmia LF, Séroussi B. Artificial intelligence in health informatics: hype or reality? Yearb Med Inform 2019;28(01):003–4.

4. Topol EJ. High-performance medicine: the convergence of human and artificial intelligence. Nat Med 2019;25(1):44–56.

5. Hood L, Flores M. A personal view on systems medicine and the emergence of proactive P4 medicine: predictive, preventive, personalized and participatory. N Biotechnol 2012;29:613–24.

6. Sriram RD. Intelligent systems for engineering - a knowledge-based approach. London: Springer Verlag; 1997. p. 1–804.

7. Russell SJ, Norvig P. Artificial intelligence: a modern approach. Third Edition. Upper Saddle River (NJ): Pearson Education Limited; 2010.

8. Sriram RD. Chapter knowledge representation. Intelligent systems for engineering. London: Springer; 1997. p. 103–58.

9. Warner H, Sorenson D, Bouhaddou O. Knowledge engineering in health informatics. New York: Springer Verlag; 1997.

10. Buchanan B, Shortliffe E. Rule-based expert systems. Reading (MA): Addison Wesley; 1984. Available at: http://www.shortliffe.net/.

11. Mitchell TM. Machine learning, vol. 45. Burr Ridge (IL): McGraw Hill; 1997. p. 870-7, 37.

12. Murphy K. Machine learning: a probabilistic perspective. Cambridge (MA): MIT Press; 2012.

13. Zubarev V. Machine learning for everyone. Available at: https://vas3k.com/blog/machine_learning/?fbclid=IwAR0f5ceCQC6v6TXg21rNdU9cvAKxNXmRtuGIqtBpIAHwsSUrFtnJpJD9nW8. Accessed January 1, 2020.

14. Kober J, Peters J. Learning motor skills: from algorithms to robot experiments. Heidelberg, Germany: Springer; 2013. Chapter 4.

15. Bishop CM. Neural networks for pattern recognition. Oxford, UK: Oxford University Press; 1995.

16. Goodfellow I, Bengio Y, Courville A. Deep learning. Cambridge (MA): MIT Press; 2016.

17. Vashist SK. Continuous glucose monitoring systems: a review. Diagnostics 2013; 3:385–412.

18. Gonzales WV, Mobashsher A, Abbosh A. The progress of glucose monitoring—a review of invasive to minimally and non-invasive techniques, devices, and sensors. Sensors 2019;19(4) [pii:E800].

19. Agrawal P, Zhong A, Phukan A, et al. Sugar. IQ insights: an innovative personalized machine-learning model for diabetes management 77th Scientific Sessions. San Diego (CA): American Diabetes Association; 2017. June 9 - 13.

20. Min W, Jiang S, Liu L, et al. A Survey on Food Computing, ACM Computing Surveys, Vol. 52, No. 5, 2019.

21. Reddy M, Pesl P, Xenou M, et al. Clinical safety and feasibility of the advanced bolus calculator for type 1 diabetes based on case-based reasoning: a 6-week nonrandomized single-arm pilot study. Diabetes Technol Ther 2016;18(8): 487–93.

22. Steil GM, Rebrin K, Darwin C, et al. Feasibility of automating insulin delivery for the treatment of type 1 diabetes. Diabetes 2006;55(12):3344–50.

23. Mauseth R, Hirsch IB, Bollyky J, et al. Use of a "fuzzy logic" controller in a closed-loop artificial pancreas. Diabetes Technol Ther 2013;15(8):628–33.

24. Weisman A, Bai JW, Cardinez M, et al. Effect of artificial pancreas systems on glycaemic control in patients with type 1 diabetes: a systematic review and meta-analysis of outpatient randomised controlled trials. Lancet Diabetes Endocrinol 2017;5(7):501–12.

25. Roychowdhury S, Koozekanani DD, Parhi KK. DREAM: diabetic retinopathy analysis using machine learning. IEEE J Biomed Health Inform 2014;18(5):1717–28.

26. Gulshan V, Peng L, Coram M, et al. Development and validation of a deep learning algorithm for detection of diabetic retinopathy in retinal fundus photographs. Jama 2016;316(22):2402–10.

27. Gargeya R, Theodore L. Automated identification of diabetic retinopathy using deep learning. Ophthalmology 2017;124(7):962–9.

28. Lam C, Yi D, Guo M, et al. Automated detection of diabetic retinopathy using deep learning. AMIA Jt Summits Transl Sci Proc 2018;2017:147–55.

29. Zeng X, Chen H, Luo Y, Ye W. Automated detection of diabetic retinopathy using a binocular siamese-like convolutional network. IEEE Access 2019;7:30744–53.

30. Zeng X, Chen H, Luo Y, Ye W. Automated detection of diabetic retinopathy using a binocular siamese-like convolutional network. 2019 IEEE International Symposium on Circuits and Systems (ISCAS), Sapporo Japan, May 26-29, 2019. p. 908–12.
31. Szegedy C, Vanhoucke V, Ioffe S, et al. Rethinking the inception architecture for computer vision. Proceedings of the IEEE conference on computer vision and pattern recognition, Las Vegas (NV), June 26-July 1, 2016. p. 2818–26.
32. Bhat TN, Collard J, Subrahmanian E, et al. Generating domain terminologies using Root- and rule-based terms. Washington Academy of Sciences Journal 2018. Winter:31–78.
33. Peleg M. Computer-interpretable clinical guidelines: a methodological review. J Biomed Inform 2013;46(4):744–63.
34. Rigla M, Martínez-Sarriegui I, García-Sáez G, et al. Gestational diabetes management using smart mobile telemedicine. J Diabetes Sci Technol 2018;12(2):260–4.
35. Grady D. A.I. Took a test to detect lung cancer. it got an A. - the New York Times. New York: New York Times; 2019. Available at: https://www.nytimes.com/2019/05/20/health/cancer-artificial-intelligence-ct-scans.html. Accessed: May 26, 2019.
36. Marcus G, Davis E. Rebooting AI: building artificial intelligence we can trust. New York: Pantheon; 2019.

Nonalcoholic Fatty Liver Disease and Implications for Older Adults with Diabetes

Alessandro Mantovani, MD, Giovanni Targher, MD,
Giacomo Zoppini, MD, PhD*

KEYWORDS

- Nonalcoholic fatty liver disease • NAFLD • Nonalcoholic steatohepatitis • NASH
- Elderly • Type 2 diabetes • Diabetes

KEY POINTS

- Nonalcoholic fatty liver disease (NAFLD) is common in older patients with type 2 diabetes.
- NAFLD is associated with an increased risk of hepatic and extrahepatic complications.
- Appropriate diagnosis and management of NAFLD are clinically relevant in older patients with diabetes.
- Specific characteristics of elderly patients (frailty, multimorbidity, and polypharmacy) should be considered.

INTRODUCTION

Nonalcoholic fatty liver disease (NAFLD) is considered the hepatic manifestation of the metabolic syndrome and comprises a spectrum of progressive pathologic conditions, spanning from simple steatosis to steatohepatitis (NASH), advanced fibrosis, cirrhosis, and, ultimately, hepatocellular cancer (HCC).[1–4] NAFLD is currently the most common chronic liver disease worldwide, affecting approximately 25% of adults in the general population,[1–4] and nearly 70% of patients with type 2 diabetes.[5,6] Importantly, patients with type 2 diabetes have a higher risk of developing the advanced forms of NAFLD,[5,6] and those with NASH or advanced fibrosis have the highest rates of liver- and non-liver-related mortality.[7–9] The early identification of this high-risk patient is fundamental to reduce the burden associated with this disease.

NAFLD occurs more often in men than in women, and, typically, affects the middle-aged and the elderly,[1–4,10] probably because the main risk factors (such as

Funding: None.
Section of Endocrinology, Diabetes, and Metabolism, University and Azienda Ospedaliera Universitaria Integrata of Verona, Verona, Italy
* Corresponding author. Section of Endocrinology, Diabetes, and Metabolism, University and Azienda Ospedaliera Universitaria, Integrata Piazzale Stefani, 1, Verona 37126, Italy.
E-mail address: giacomo.zoppini@univr.it

overweight/obesity, type 2 diabetes, dyslipidemia, and sedentary lifestyle) implicated in its development and progression tend to grow in prevalence with advancing age.[10] The higher prevalence of NAFLD associated with older age may have further clinical implications.[10] First, in the elderly, NAFLD is expected to carry a relevant burden of NASH, cirrhosis, and HCC.[10] Second, when compared with those without liver involvement, elderly patients with NAFLD have an increased risk of developing specific geriatric conditions, such as sarcopenia, frailty, and dementia.[10] For these reasons, appropriate diagnosis and management of NAFLD in elderly have become a major task for clinical geriatricians and geriatric hepatologists.

In this review, the authors discuss the epidemiology of NAFLD in older patients with and without type 2 diabetes as well as the hepatic and extrahepatic complications associated with NAFLD in this patient group. Last, the authors briefly discuss the principles of NAFLD management in the elderly.

EPIDEMIOLOGY OF NONALCOHOLIC FATTY LIVER DISEASE: ROLES OF AGE AND TYPE 2 DIABETES

The prevalence of NAFLD has increased over the last 20 years[1–4] and is expected to increase exponentially in the next decade.[11] The diagnosis of NAFLD is currently based on the following criteria: (a) hepatic steatosis on imaging or histology, (b) no excessive alcohol consumption (a threshold of 20 g/d for women and 30 g/d for men is conventionally adopted), and (c) no other causes for hepatic steatosis.[12,13] In addition to the "gold-standard" diagnostic test of liver biopsy, several noninvasive techniques are available to date, in order to detect NAFLD in clinical practice. Liver ultrasonography, computed tomography (CT), and magnetic resonance are broadly accepted modalities for detecting hepatic fat content in both clinical and research settings.[12,13]

As reported in **Table 1**, several observational studies[14–22] and some metaanalyses[4,6] have investigated the prevalence of NAFLD (as detected by imaging or biopsy) in individuals with age ≥65 years. As mentioned above, aging increases the prevalence of NAFLD as well as the risk of its advanced forms, but this seems to be reliable in the time span ranging from 30 to 65 years.[23] In fact, among age groups over 65 years, the prevalence of NAFLD reaches a plateau, and substantial differences are not observed.[23] In addition, in a recent study using the Markov model to predict the progression of NAFLD, it was estimated that the ratio of male-to-female prevalence may vary by age group, with the lowest male-to-female ratio among individuals less than 30 years and the highest among individuals aged 40 to 49 years.[23]

In a US observational study of 3227 individuals, Golabi and colleagues[22] documented that the prevalence rates from NAFLD (as detected by the US Fatty Liver Index) were 40.3% and 39.2% among 60 to 74 and older than 75 year olds, respectively, indicating that NAFLD is common among the elderly population, but that no substantial difference in its prevalence exists among specific advanced age subgroup (ie, 60–74 vs >75 year olds). Similarly, in the Rotterdam study, the prevalence of NAFLD (on ultrasonography) was partly attenuated by advancing age, ranging from ~36% of participants less than 70 years to ~21% of participants aged ≥85 years.[19] In that study, the association between number of metabolic syndrome criteria and probability of NAFLD was also partly weakened with advancing age.[19]

Based on the National Health and Nutrition Examination Survey (NHANES) III data, Lazo and colleagues[21] showed that in men the peak prevalence of NAFLD (on ultrasonography) was between the ages of 50 to 60 years, with 16% in ages 30 to 40 years

Table 1
Main observational studies that have investigated the prevalence of nonalcoholic fatty liver disease in patients older than 65 years

Author, Ref.	Study Population	NAFLD Diagnosis	Main Findings
Kagansky et al,[14] *Liver Int* 2004;24:588–594	Prospective study: 91 Israeli octogenarians (mean age 85 y) who were admitted to the rehabilitation departments of a geriatric hospital	Liver ultrasonography	The prevalence of NAFLD was 46.2%
Park et al,[15] *J Gastroenterol Hepatol* 2006;21:138–143	Cross-sectional study: 6648 Korean individuals	Liver ultrasonography	Prevalence of NAFLD increased from 2.1% among women aged 20–29 y, to 10.3% for women aged 40–49 y, and spiked once age exceeded 50 y. The prevalence in men who were younger than 50 y of age was higher than that seen in women (22.6% vs 6.8%), whereas results in participants older than 50 y of age were similar (23.6% vs 24.2%)
Karnikowski et al,[16] *Sao Paulo Med J* 2007;125:333–337	Population-based study: 139 Brazilian individuals aged 55 y or older (mean age 67 y)	Liver ultrasonography	The prevalence of NAFLD was 35.2%
Frith et al,[17] *Gerontology* 2009;55:607–613	Retrospective cohort study: 351 UK consecutive patients with biopsy-proven NAFLD were divided into an older (≥60 y), a middle-aged (from ≥50 to <60 y), and a younger (<50 y) group	Liver biopsy	The prevalence of NAFLD was higher in the middle aged and in the elderly
Mantovani et al,[18] *J Endocrinol Invest* 2012;35:215–218	Cross-sectional study: 116 Italian consecutive patients with hypertension and type 2 diabetes (mean age 68 y)	Liver ultrasonography	The prevalence of NAFLD was 70%

(continued on next page)

Table 1
(continued)

Author, Ref.	Study Population	NAFLD Diagnosis	Main Findings
Koehler et al,[19] *J Hepatol* 2012;57:1305–1311	Population-based Rotterdam Study: 2811 European participants (mean age 76 y)	Liver ultrasonography	The prevalence of NAFLD ranged from 35.8% of participants <70 y to 21.1% of participants aged ≥85 y
Noureddin et al,[20] *Hepatology* 2013;58:1644–1654	Cross-sectional study: 796 US participants from the NASH Clinical Research Network study, of whom 61 were elderly (≥65 y)	Liver biopsy	Compared with nonelderly patients with NAFLD, elderly patients had a higher prevalence of NASH (56% vs 72%, $P = .02$), and advanced fibrosis (25% vs 44%, $P = .002$)
Lazo et al,[21] *Am J Epidemiol* 2013;178:38–45	Cross-sectional study: 12,454 US adults from the Third NHANES, conducted in the United States from 1988 to 1994	Liver ultrasonography	In men, the prevalence of NAFLD was 16% in ages 30–40 y old, 22% in 41–50 y old, 29% in 51–60 y old, and 28% in older than 60 y old. In women, the prevalence of NAFLD was 12% in ages 30–40 y old, 16% in 41–50 y old, 22% in 51–60 y old, and 25% in older than 60 y old
Younossi et al,[4] *Hepatology* 2016;64:73–84	Metaanalysis: 86 eligible studies with a sample size of 8,515,431 with and without type 2 diabetes	Imaging or liver biopsy	The prevalence rates of NAFLD were 27.4% (95% CI: 19.6%–36.9%) among 50–59 y, 28.9% (95% CI: 19.2%–40.9%) among 60–69 y, and 33.9% (95% CI: 32.1%–35.9%) among 70–79 y
Golabi et al,[22] *BMC Gastroenterol* 2019;19:56	Cross-sectional study: 3271 US participants from the from the Third NHANES	US Fatty Liver Index	The prevalence rates from NAFLD were 40.3% (95% CI: 37.2%–43.5%) and 39.2% (95% CI: 34.4%–44.0%) among individuals 60–74 and >74 y
Younossi et al,[6] *J Hepatol* 2019;71:793–801	Metaanalysis: 80 studies with a total of 49,419 individuals with established type 2 diabetes	Imaging or liver biopsy	The prevalence of imaging-diagnosed NAFLD was 56.4% among individuals <50 y, 56.5% among individuals 50–59 y, and 62.8% among those ≥60 y

old, 22% in 41 to 50 years old, 29% in 51 to 60 years old, and 28% in those older than 60 years old. In women, instead, the prevalence of NAFLD increased with age especially after menopause, with 12% in ages 30 to 40 years old, 16% in 41 to 50 years old, 22% in 51 to 60 years old, and 25% in those older than 60 years old.[21] Interestingly, in a small observational study involving 91 octogenarians (mean age 85 ± 4 years), who were admitted to rehabilitation departments of a geriatric hospital, Kagansky and colleagues[14] documented that the prevalence of NAFLD, as detected by ultrasonography, was approximately 46%.

Different findings were partly observed among Asian patients. In a cross-sectional study involving 6648 Korean individuals, the prevalence of NAFLD (on ultrasonography) increased with age only among women, whereas its prevalence in men differed little across all age groups.[15] In that study, the aforementioned observed gaps between age groups and gender may be explained by the relatively high prevalence of obesity among men younger than 50 years of age.[15] In a cross-sectional study of 2782 Bangladeshi participants, Alam and colleagues[24] reported that the prevalence of NAFLD increases with advanced age, with almost similar prevalence in ages 45 to 54 and in ages ≥55 years.

These findings were also confirmed in a metaanalysis of 86 eligible studies with a sample size of nearly 9,000,000 individuals with and without type 2 diabetes.[4] In that study, Younossi and colleagues[4] reported that the prevalence rates of imaging-diagnosed NAFLD were 27.4% (95% confidence interval [CI]: 19.6%–36.9%) among 50 to 59 year olds, 28.9% (95% CI: 19.2%–40.9%) among 60 to 69 year olds, and 33.9% (95% CI: 32.1%–35.9%) among 70 to 79 year olds. Of note, recently, in another metaanalysis of 80 studies with a total of 49,419 individuals with established type 2 diabetes, it was documented that the prevalence of imaging-diagnosed NAFLD was ~56% among individuals less than 50 years, ~57% among individuals 50 to 59 years, and ~63% among those ≥60 years.[6]

The differences in NAFLD prevalence among various age groups may be explained, at least in part, by the fact that the main risk factors involved in the development and progression of NAFLD tend to increase in prevalence with advancing age. In fact, in addition to age, NAFLD has been shown to be independently associated with type 2 diabetes and metabolic syndrome.[25,26] Studies that used liver biopsy for diagnosing NAFLD reported that the prevalence of NASH and advanced fibrosis among patients with type 2 diabetes were 70% and 30% to 40%, respectively, thus exceeding that of the general population.[27] For instance, in a large cohort study of 1249 US patients with biopsy-proven NAFLD, the prevalence of NASH and advanced fibrosis in patients with type 2 diabetes were 69% and 41%, respectively.[28] In some biopsy studies, it has also emerged that the development of incidence of type 2 diabetes was the strongest predictor of progression to NASH and liver fibrosis.[27,29] Indeed, in a study of nearly 1100 diabetic and nondiabetic patients with histological-proven NAFLD from the PIVENS trial and the NAFLD Database Study, Loomba and colleagues[30] documented that the presence of both established type 2 diabetes and family history of diabetes were strong and independent predictors of NASH and advanced fibrosis on liver histology. In another study of 235 patients with biopsy-proven NAFLD, Puchakayala and colleagues[31] reported that patients with type 2 diabetes had a higher NAFLD activity score and higher fibrosis score when compared with those without type 2 diabetes. In addition, in that study, patients with type 2 diabetes had a significantly higher prevalence of advanced fibrosis and ballooning when compared with those without type 2 diabetes. Notably, poor glycemic control may also increase the risk of fibrosis in NASH.[31]

NONALCOHOLIC FATTY LIVER DISEASE AND MAIN GERIATRIC SYNDROMES: SARCOPENIA, FRAILTY, AND DEMENTIA

The association between NAFLD and some clinical syndromes typically associated with aging (including sarcopenia, frailty, and dementia) is still scarcely defined to date.

Sarcopenia and Frailty

Sarcopenia is characterized by reduced muscle mass and strength as well as replacement of muscle with adipose and fibrous tissue.[32,33] Sarcopenia may lead to functional impairment, physical disability, frailty, and even mortality.[32,33] Importantly, its prevalence continues to increase worldwide, probably as a result of increased elderly populations.[32,33] The most commonly used, low-cost, and accessible methods to assess sarcopenia are dual-energy X-ray absorptiometry, anthropometry, and bioelectrical impedance analysis. Other methods include MRI and CT.[33]

As shown in **Table 2**,[34–42] some cross-sectional studies[34–39,41,42] and a metaanalysis[40] have recently documented that sarcopenia is associated with NAFLD and its advanced forms in patients with and without type 2 diabetes. These associations seem to remain even after adjustment for several metabolic confounders, such as obesity and insulin resistance. For instance, in a cross-sectional study involving 225 Italian consecutive patients with biopsy-proven NAFLD, Petta and colleagues[38] showed that the prevalence of sarcopenia (as detected by weight-adjusted appendicular skeletal muscle mass) increased with the severity of hepatic fibrosis. In addition, in that study, the multivariate analysis documented that sarcopenia was significantly associated with the severity of hepatic fibrosis and steatosis, independent of multiple metabolic confounders.

In a cross-sectional study of 2761 Korean individuals with NAFLD from Korean National Health and Nutrition Examination Surveys 2008-2011, Lee and colleagues[36] documented that sarcopenia (as detected by dual-energy X-ray absorptiometry) was independently associated with an increased risk of advanced liver fibrosis, evaluated indirectly by noninvasive markers (ie, FIB-4 score and NAFLD fibrosis score), even after adjustment for age, body mass index, waist circumference, insulin resistance, fasting glucose, lipids, liver enzymes, diabetes, hypertension, exercise, smoking, kidney function, drinking, and prior history of cerebrovascular and coronary heart disease, chronic obstructive pulmonary disease, and malignancy. In another study of 309 Asian individuals with and without biopsy-proven NAFLD, the prevalence of sarcopenia (measured by weight-adjusted appendicular skeletal muscle mass) in patients without NAFLD, with nonalcoholic fatty liver, and with NASH were approximately 9%, 18%, and 35%, respectively. Interestingly, in that study, sarcopenia was significantly associated with both NASH and significant fibrosis, independent of age, gender, body mass index, hypertension, diabetes, smoking status, and insulin resistance.[39] These findings were also confirmed in a recent metaanalysis of 6 cross-sectional studies for a total of nearly 16,000 individuals with and without type 2 diabetes.[40]

In addition, recently, in a study of 3969 Chinese adults, Xia and colleagues[41] reported the existence of an association between sarcopenia and NAFLD only in patatin-like phospholipase domain-containing 3 (PNPLA3) CC and CG genotype carriers. A dissociation of sarcopenia and NAFLD was, instead, observed in PNPLA3 GG genotype carriers, thereby suggesting that a stratification based on PNPLA3 genotypes might additionally help the development of a personalized management for NAFLD patients.[41]

Table 2
Principal observational studies and metaanalysis investigating the association between sarcopenia and nonalcoholic fatty liver disease (ordered by publication data)

Author, Ref.	Study Population	NAFLD Diagnosis	Sarcopenia Diagnosis	Statistical Adjustment	Main Findings
Hong et al,[34] *Hepatology* 2014;59:1772–1778	Cross-sectional study: 452 apparently healthy adults enrolled in the Korean Sarcopenic Obesity Study	CT	The skeletal muscle index	Age, sex	Sarcopenia was associated with increased risks of NAFLD
Lee et al,[35] *J Hepatol* 2015;63:486–493.	Cross-sectional study: 15,132 individuals from the Korea National Health and Nutrition Examination Surveys 2008–2011	NAFLD score or NAFLD liver fat score and indirect markers of advanced fibrosis (ie, BARD, FIB-4 score)	The skeletal muscle index	Age, sex, regular exercise, HOMA-IR, smoking, hypertension	Sarcopenia was associated with increased risks of NAFLD and advanced fibrosis
Lee et al,[36] *Hepatology* 2016;63:776–786	Cross-sectional study: 2761 Korean individuals with NAFLD from Korean National Health and Nutrition Examination Surveys 2008-2011	NAFLD liver fat score and indirect markers of advanced fibrosis (ie, NAFLD Fibrosis Score, FIB-4 score)	Sarcopenia index	Age, body mass index, waist circumference, insulin resistance, glucose, lipids, liver enzymes, diabetes, hypertension, exercise, smoking, kidney function, drinking, prior history of cerebrovascular and coronary heart disease, chronic obstructive pulmonary disease, malignancy	Sarcopenia was associated with liver fibrosis in individuals with NAFLD

(continued on next page)

Table 2
(continued)

Author, Ref.	Study Population	NAFLD Diagnosis	Sarcopenia Diagnosis	Statistical Adjustment	Main Findings
Hashimoto et al,[37] *Endocr J* 2016;63:877–884	Cross-sectional study: 145 Japanese patients with type 2 diabetes	Ultrasonography and controlled attenuation parameter	The skeletal muscle index	Age, BMI, hemoglobin A1c, triglycerides/HDL-C ratio, C-reactive protein, gamma-glutamyl transferase	Sarcopenia was associated with an increased risk of NAFLD in men, but not in women
Petta et al,[38] *Aliment Pharmacol Ther* 2017;45:510–518	Cross-sectional study: 225 Italian consecutive patients with histologic diagnosis of NAFLD	Liver biopsy	The skeletal muscle index	Age, gender, BMI, obesity, alanine aminotransferase, triglycerides, glucose, insulin, diabetes, hypertension, medications	Sarcopenia was associated with the severity of fibrosis and steatosis
Koo et al,[39] *J Hepatol* 2017;66:123–131	Cross-sectional study: 309 Korean individuals with and without biopsy-proven NAFLD	Liver biopsy	Weight-adjusted appendicular skeletal muscle mass	Age, gender, BMI, hypertension, diabetes, smoking status, and insulin resistance	Sarcopenia was associated with NASH and significant fibrosis
Pan et al,[40] *Dig Dis* 2018;36:427–436	Metaanalysis: 6 eligible studies for a total of approximately 16,000 individuals	Imaging, liver biopsy	The skeletal muscle index; weight-adjusted appendicular skeletal muscle mass	Multiple cardiometabolic confounders	Sarcopenia was associated with NAFLD and significant fibrosis

Xia et al,[41] *Aliment Pharmacol Ther* 2019;50:684–695	Cross-sectional study: 3969 Chinese adults	Ultrasonography and indirect markers of advanced fibrosis (ie, NAFLD Fibrosis Score, BARD, FIB-4 score)	Weight-adjusted appendicular skeletal muscle mass	Age, cigarette smoking, fat mass, obesity, diabetes, metabolic syndrome	The association between sarcopenia and NAFLD was observed only in PNPLA3 CC and CG genotype carriers
Chung et al,[42] *J Obes Metab Syndr* 2019; 28:129–138	Cross-sectional study: 5989 Korean individuals	Ultrasonography	Weight-adjusted appendicular skeletal muscle mass	Age, sex, visceral fat area, hypertension, diabetes, total and low-density lipoprotein cholesterol	Sarcopenia was associated with increased risk of NAFLD

Abbreviations: BMI, body mass index; HDL-C, high-density lipoprotein cholesterol; HOMA-IR, homeostasis model assessment of insulin resistance.

Collectively, these findings suggest that sarcopenia is independently associated with NAFLD in individuals with and without type 2 diabetes. In the interpretation of these data, one must however note that, first, most studies were conducted in Asian individuals, and second, the methods used for the diagnosis of NAFLD and sarcopenia vary across cross-sectional studies. Third, no longitudinal studies with an adequate follow-up are available to date.

Sarcopenia and NAFLD share several pathophysiologic mechanisms that may partly explain the associations observed in the aforementioned studies.[34–42] First, insulin resistance has been consistently associated with both conditions.[10,32] The relationship between insulin resistance and NAFLD is well established.[5,43] The skeletal muscle is one of the main tissues responsible for insulin-mediated glucose disposal, and the prominent role of skeletal muscle in insulin resistance has been confirmed by several epidemiologic and experimental studies.[10,32,33] In some observational studies (for example in the study of Koo and colleagues[39]), the association between NAFLD and sarcopenia was partly attenuated by the adjustment for Homeostatic Model Assessment of Insulin Resistanc, suggesting that such association might be mediated, at least in part, by insulin resistance.[10,32,33] Second, inflammation may be also an important link between sarcopenia and NAFLD.[10,32,34–42] Low muscle mass is associated with chronic inflammation and, on the other hand, subclinical inflammation and oxidative stress promote the catabolic stimulation of muscle resulting in the loss of muscle mass.[10,32,33] Oxidative stress and chronic inflammation are also important factors in the development and progression of NAFLD.[5,43] In this regard, it is important to highlight that in some observational studies (for example, in the study of Koo and colleagues[39]), the association between sarcopenia and NAFLD was slightly attenuated after adjustment for highly sensitive C-reactive protein levels, thereby suggesting that chronic inflammation might be a potential mediator of 2 conditions. Third, accumulating evidence now reports that low vitamin D levels may be associated with sarcopenia and with NAFLD.[10,32,40] In the Longitudinal Aging Study Amsterdam, Visser and colleagues[44] reported the existence of an association between lower levels of 25-OH vitamin D and lower muscle mass. In addition, other studies reported that in individuals with vitamin D deficiency, there are histologic alterations of muscle composition and diameter and that supplementation of 25[OH]D may have some beneficial effects.[10,33,44] Similarly, observational studies have documented a lower level of vitamin D in patients with NAFLD.[10,45] Experimental evidence suggests that 25[OH]D may interfere with the activation of hepatic stellate cells that are involved in the development of hepatic fibrosis.[10,45]

Dementia

Cognitive decline is a pathologic feature of aging and diabetes.[10,46] In the last decade, experimental and observational data have suggested the existence of an independent association between NAFLD (as detected by imaging or biopsy) and impaired cognitive function.[10] For instance, in an experimental study conducted in rats with and without NAFLD, Ghareeb and colleagues[47] documented that liver steatohepatitis induced important alterations in neurotransmitter activities, concurring to the development of brain dysfunction and tissue damage. In another experimental study conducted in mice with and without NAFLD, Kim and colleagues[48] showed that the systemic chronic inflammation induced by NAFLD induced neuroinflammation and neurodegeneration in the brain of these animals, leading to neuronal death in cortical and hippocampal areas. Interestingly, when the investigators removed mice from a high-fat diet regimen, they observed a reduction of neuroinflammatory and neurodegenerative along with an improvement of liver steatosis.[48]

Despite these and other experimental data, clinical evidence on cognitive functioning in patients with NAFLD is still limited to date. In an observational study involving 224 patients with biopsy-proven NAFLD and 107 patients with biopsy-proven alcoholic liver disease (ALD) who performed validated functional, cognitive, autonomic, and fatigue symptom assessment tools at baseline and after 3 years of follow-up, Elliott and colleagues[49] documented that NAFLD and ALD patients had functional impairment affecting activities of daily living when compared with healthy controls. In a cross-sectional study including approximately 4500 adults from the Third National Health and Nutritional Examination Survey of Korea who underwent cognitive evaluation using the validated computer-administered tests (ie, Simple Reaction Time Test, the Symbol-Digit Substitution Test, and the Serial Digit Learning Test), Seo and colleagues[50] documented that patients with NAFLD (on ultrasonography) had a lower cognitive performance, when compared with those without NAFLD. In addition, in another cross-sectional study of 70 individuals with NAFLD (on ultrasonography) and 73 age- and sex-matched healthy controls who performed the Montreal Cognitive Assessment, Celikbilek and colleagues[51] showed that patients with NAFLD had cognitive dysfunction more frequently, especially in the visuospatial and executive function domains, when compared with controls. Interestingly, in a study of 40 patients with NAFLD and 36 controls, Filipoviç and colleagues[52] documented that patients with NAFLD had lower brain tissue volumes (on MRI) when compared with those without liver involvement. Similar findings were also observed in the offspring cohort of the Framingham Study[53] and in the CARDIA study.[54] This evidence may suggest an association between NAFLD and a smaller total cerebral brain volume, indicating a potential link between liver steatosis and brain aging. To date, information regarding different cognitive function risk in relation to NAFLD severity is still scarce. Recently, in a cross-sectional study involving 1287 adults, Weinstein and colleagues[55] reported that the presence of NAFLD (as detected by CT) was not associated with cognitive function, evaluated by cognitive testing of memory, abstract reasoning, visual perception, attention, and executive function. However, when the investigators restricted the analyses exclusively to patients with NAFLD, they observed that those with advanced fibrosis (as detected by NAFLD fibrosis score) had poorer cognitive performance, when compared with those without advanced fibrosis.[55]

The pathologic mechanisms linking NAFLD and measures of cognitive function are not fully understood. Seeing that most studies have found an association between NAFLD and executive function (that reflects the integrity of the frontal lobe[53–55]) and that NAFLD is strongly associated with vascular alterations,[56–58] it is possible to speculate that an important underlying mechanism of this association may be the subclinical vascular injury. Other explanations for the association between NAFLD and poor cognitive function may include oxidative stress, insulin resistance, and the secretion of cytokines that may contribute to the development of chronic inflammatory and fibrotic processes.[46,56–58]

HEPATIC COMPLICATIONS OF NONALCOHOLIC FATTY LIVER DISEASE IN THE GERIATRIC AGE GROUP

As mentioned above, NAFLD has become a significant cause of cirrhosis, end-stage liver disease, and liver transplantation.[1–4,59,60] However, only a small proportion of individuals with NAFLD progress to cirrhosis and develop liver-related morbidity.[59,60]

Analogously to other chronic liver diseases, the severity of underlying liver fibrosis is an important marker of adverse outcome, with patients with bridging fibrosis or cirrhosis being at greatest risk of future liver- and non-liver-related morbidity.[7–9,59,60]

Recently, in a longitudinal study involving 475 patients with NASH and bridging fibrosis or compensated cirrhosis followed for a total of 96 weeks, Sanyal and colleagues[59] documented a high proportion of patients (~22%) that developed serious liver-related complications. Similarly, in 2003, Hui and colleagues[61] found a 23% incidence of decompensation at 3 years in a small cohort of patients with NASH cirrhosis. Although NASH is thought to be a slowly progressive disease, this aspect suggests the presence of heterogeneity in disease progression with a subset of patients having an accelerated disease course.[59,60] These findings are also supported by a recent metaanalysis of NAFLD patients undergoing liver biopsies, documenting that a relatively high proportion of patients (~21%) developed F3/4 fibrosis from a baseline of no fibrosis over a mean follow-up of ~6 years.[62]

Risk factors for HCC and liver-related mortality in patients with NAFLD include advanced age, type 2 diabetes, and cirrhosis.[63] Notably, HCC may also develop in patients with noncirrhotic NAFLD.[63] In the elderly, decreased cytochrome P450 activity may affect drug metabolism, thus favoring the drug-related liver injury.[10] Immune responses against pathogens or neoplastic cells tend to be reduced in the elderly.[10] Hence, alterations in immune functions may alter the pathogenesis of viral hepatitis and autoimmune liver diseases as well as the development of HCC.[10]

EXTRAHEPATIC COMPLICATIONS OF NONALCOHOLIC FATTY LIVER DISEASE IN THE GERIATRIC AGE GROUP: SPOTLIGHT ON CARDIOVASCULAR DISEASE

In the last decade, several observational studies have documented that NAFLD (as detected by imaging) is independently associated with an increased risk of fatal and nonfatal cardiovascular events in patients with and without diabetes.[58] In particular, accumulating evidence now suggests that NAFLD adversely affects not only the coronary arteries (thereby promoting accelerated coronary atherosclerosis) but also all other anatomic structures of the heart, leading to an increased risk of cardiomyopathy (eg, left ventricular diastolic dysfunction and hypertrophy), cardiac valvular calcification (eg, aortic-valve sclerosis and mitral annulus calcification), cardiac arrhythmias (eg, atrial fibrillation), and some cardiac conduction defects.[57] Notably, these findings tend to be common in the elderly.[57]

With regard to atrial fibrillation (which is the most frequent arrhythmia observed in clinical practice and is strongly associated with high rates of hospitalization and death), it is known that the prevalence of atrial fibrillation increases from 1% in individuals less than 55 years of age to 12% in those older than 80 years of age.[57,64] Along with older age, obesity, hypertension, coronary heart disease, heart failure, and heart valve disease are the other important risk factors for new-onset atrial fibrillation.[64] NAFLD is associated with multiple abnormalities in cardiac structure and function and shares multiple cardiometabolic risk factors with atrial fibrillation. An association between NAFLD and an increased risk of incident atrial fibrillation in type 2 diabetic patients older than 60 years has been reported.[65] Similar findings have been confirmed in other observational studies and some recent metaanalyses.[57,66,67] Accumulating evidence has reported the existence of an independent association between NAFLD and risk of QTc prolongation, which is strongly related to the development of serious cardiac arrhythmias. In a cross-sectional study of approximately 32,000 Korean adults, Hung and colleagues[57,68,69] found that NAFLD (on ultrasonography) was associated with an increased risk of QTc prolongation, independent of multiple cardiovascular risk factors. Interestingly, a relationship between NAFLD and risk of ventricular arrhythmias has also been documented.[57] In a cross-sectional study of 330 Italian outpatients with type 2 diabetes who performed a clinically indicated 24-hour ambulatory Holter monitoring,

Mantovani and colleagues[70] reported that NAFLD (as detected by ultrasonography) was associated with an increased risk of ventricular arrhythmias, independent of several confounding factors. In addition, preliminary data support a relationship between NAFLD and cardiac conduction defects, which are strong independent predictors of all-cause and cardiovascular mortality.[57,71]

With regard to heart valve calcification, it is important to highlight that aortic valve sclerosis (AVS) and mitral annular calcification (MAC) are common echocardiographic findings in the elderly, occurring in up to 20%.[57] Observational studies have reported an association between imaging-diagnosed NAFLD and risk of AVS and MAC in patients with and without type 2 diabetes.[72,73]

Accumulating evidence also suggests that NAFLD is associated with functional and structural myocardial abnormalities in adult individuals with and without type 2 diabetes.[57] For instance, in a cross-sectional study involving 222 consecutive type 2 diabetic outpatients with no previous history of ischemic heart disease, chronic heart failure, valvular diseases, and known hepatic diseases, Mantovani and colleagues[74] documented that NAFLD was associated with a 3-fold increased risk of mild and/or moderate left ventricular diastolic dysfunction (on echocardiography) even after adjusting for age, sex, body mass index, hypertension, diabetes duration, hemoglobin A1c, estimated glomerular filtration rate, left ventricular mass index, and ejection fraction. In another cross-sectional study of 116 consecutive elderly patients with hypertension and type 2 diabetes, it was documented that NAFLD was associated with left ventricular hypertrophy independent of classical cardiovascular risk factors and other potential confounders.[18] Other studies, using biopsy-proven NAFLD, have found a direct, graded relationship between functional and structural myocardial abnormalities and the severity of NAFLD.[57]

MANAGEMENT OF NONALCOHOLIC FATTY LIVER DISEASE IN THE GERIATRIC AGE GROUP

To date, there are no approved pharmacologic treatments for NAFLD and its advanced forms in adult patients with and without type 2 diabetes.[12,13,57] The NAFLD management essentially focuses on 4 of the following key goals: (a) lifestyle change in order to effect weight loss and reduce obesity; (b) control of the cardiometabolic risk factors, using agents with potential beneficial liver effects; (c) correction of all modifiable factors that lead to the development and progression of liver fibrosis (seeing that the hepatic fibrosis appears to be the strongest predictor of poor long-term outcomes); and (d) prevention of both hepatic and extrahepatic complications.[12,13,57,75] Hence, interventions addressing obesity and the features of metabolic syndrome (ie, dyslipidemia, hypertension, impaired fasting glucose) may exert advantageous effects on the risk of NAFLD-related complications.[12,13,57,75] However, it is important to note that no intervention on NAFLD has been assessed in elderly patients, because most studies published so far have recruited only middle-aged individuals.

Nonpharmacologic treatment should be individually tailored considering the physical limitations of most elderly people and the necessity for an adequate caloric supply in most cases.[10,75] All patients with NAFLD, independent of the presence of diabetes, should avoid cigarette smoking and consumption of alcohol as well as of fructose-containing beverages and foods.[12,13,57]

Probably, for the reasons mentioned above, pharmacotherapy for NAFLD should be reserved for patients with NASH and advanced fibrosis.[12,13,57,76] To date, however, there are very few high-quality, randomized, blinded, adequately powered, controlled studies of sufficient duration and with adequate histologic outcomes conducted in patients with and without type 2 diabetes.[12,13,57,76] The most consistence data for the treatment of NAFLD concern the use of pioglitazone in patients with biopsy-proven NASH.[12,13,76] Pioglitazone is a selective ligand of the peroxisome-proliferator–activated receptor-gamma and is able to ameliorate glucose and lipid metabolism and also to reduce subclinical inflammation.[76,77] Several studies documented that pioglitazone improves liver histology, including steatosis and necroinflammation in patients with and without type 2 diabetes.[76] In this context, in a randomized, double-blind, placebo-controlled trial of approximately 100 middle-aged patients with prediabetes or type 2 diabetes and biopsy-proven NASH randomly assigned to pioglitazone or placebo, Cusi and colleagues[78] reported that, among the pioglitazone arm, more than half of the patients achieved the primary study outcome (described as a reduction of at least 2 points in the NAFLD activity score without worsening of fibrosis), and half of them also had a resolution of NASH over a period of 18 months. In addition, in a recent metaanalysis of 8 randomized controlled trials for a total of nearly 520 patients with biopsy-proven NASH, Musso and colleagues[79] reported that pioglitazone was associated with improved advanced fibrosis and NASH resolution over a period of treatment ranging from 6 to 24 months. In this regard, pioglitazone may be considered for treatment in biopsy-proven NASH, also according to American Association for the Study of Liver Diseases and European Association for the Study of Liver guidelines.[12,13] However, it is important to underline that pioglitazone is not approved by most agencies outer the treatment of type 2 diabetes, and its off-label use for NAFLD always needs the patient's consent.[76] In addition, concerns about weight gain, fluid retention, bone fractures, and risk of bladder cancer may partly restrict the use of pioglitazone.[77] Seeing that patients with NAFLD have an increased risk of cardiovascular disease and chronic kidney disease when compared with those without,[57,58] it is also important to remember that pioglitazone exerts cardiovascular benefits in patients with and without type 2 diabetes,[80,81] thereby making this glucose-lowering agent somewhat appealing for the treatment of NAFLD.

Metformin is an insulin sensitizer and, to date, is broadly considered the first-line therapeutic agent for the treatment of type 2 diabetes.[76,77] Metformin reduces blood glucose levels by mechanisms involving an AMP-activated protein kinase–dependent improvement of hepatic glucose metabolism and increased glucose uptake into muscle cells.[76,77] Several studies have documented that metformin, despite its beneficial effects on liver enzymes, HbA1c levels, and other metabolic parameters, had a neutral effect on liver histology and resolution of NASH in adults.[76] Consequently, to date, the US and the European guidelines for NAFLD do not support the use of metformin for the treatment of NAFLD.[12,13] That said, it is also important to underline that, currently, the potential advantages of metformin in chronic liver disease (in adult patients with or without type 2 diabetes) may be restricted to its effect in reducing the risk of cirrhosis and hepatocellular carcinoma.[63]

The incretin mimetic drugs (ie, dipeptidyl peptidase [DPP]-4 inhibitors and glucagon-like peptide [GLP]-1 receptor agonists) are broadly prescribed as additional therapy in patients with type 2 diabetes.[76,77] These glucose-lowering agents are effective for the treatment of type 2 diabetes and may improve insulin sensitivity.[76,77] It is important to highlight that GLP-1 receptors have been documented in human hepatocytes and that the activation of these receptors may favor the reduction of hepatic steatosis by improving insulin signaling.[76] In addition, GLP-1R agonists can help to promote weight loss.[77] Based on these data, GLP-1R agonists have been investigated as a therapeutic option for NAFLD. Several studies support the capability of GLP-1R agonists to reduce plasma aminotransferases (especially alanine aminotransferase) and improve hepatic steatosis, as detected by imaging techniques or histology.[82–84]

In particular, liraglutide was tested in middle-aged NASH patients by the LEAD (Lira-glutide Effect and Action in Diabetes) program[82] and the LEAN trial,[84] with significant benefit in several metabolic and hepatic end points, such as peripheral, hepatic, and adipose tissue insulin resistance, resolution of NASH, and improvement of steatosis and ballooning. However, no information is available to date in patients older than 65 years. Importantly, liraglutide has been shown to reduce cardiovascular events in patients with type 2 diabetes in the LEADER trial[85] and in a recent metaanalysis.[86]

DPP-4 inhibitors block DPP-4 enzyme, thus preventing the inactivation of incretins (ie, glucose-dependent insulinotropic polypeptide and GLP-1).[76,77] By this effect, DPP-4 inhibitors may stimulate insulin secretion, lower hepatic glucose output, and suppress glucagon release. Moreover, when compared with those without NAFLD, in-dividuals with NAFLD have a higher expression of DPP-4 in the liver.[76,77] For this reason, DPP-4 inhibitors have been investigated as a therapeutic option for NAFLD.[76,77] As one of the earliest commercially available DPP-4 inhibitors, sitagliptin has been broadly used to assess efficacy of DPP-4 inhibitors in patients with NAFLD. In a 24-week randomized, double-blind, placebo-controlled trial of NAFLD patients with impaired glucose tolerance or type 2 diabetes, Cui and colleagues[87] documented no statistically difference in liver fat content (as detected by MRI–proton density fat fraction) between sitagliptin and placebo. Notably, DPP-4 inhibitors appear to have a neutral effect on cardiovascular outcomes in patients with type 2 diabetes,[88] thereby making this class of glucose-lowering agents not attractive for the treatment of NAFLD.

Sodium glucose co-transporter 2 (SGLT-2) inhibitors are a new class of oral hypo-glycemic agents that play by decreasing renal glucose reabsorption.[76,77] Experimental studies support a protective effect of SGLT-2 inhibitors on hepatic steatosis, inflam-mation, and fibrosis, probably because of a combination of negative energy balance by glycosuria and substrate switching toward lipids as a source of energy expendi-ture.[89] Several studies support the assertion that SGLT-2 inhibitors may determine a reduction of hepatic fat content, as evaluated by MRI or CT.[89] A reduction in trans-aminase levels was also documented.[89] However, no specific study in elderly patients has been conducted so far.

Seeing that increased oxidative stress occurs in both NAFLD and type 2 diabetes, another therapeutic option for NAFLD treatment may be to decrease oxidative stress by administration of vitamin E.[57,76,90] In the PIVENS trial, involving approximately 250 nondiabetic adults with NASH, the treatment with vitamin E for 96 weeks, when compared with placebo, was associated with improvements in liver enzymes and his-tologic features of NASH, including steatosis, inflammation, and ballooning.[90] Howev-er, insufficient evidence is available to treat older patients with diabetes or cirrhosis.

Pentoxifylline is able to decrease oxidative stress and inhibit lipid oxidation.[90] Several studies have documented that pentoxifylline can decrease in serum liver en-zymes and improve steatosis, lobular inflammation, and fibrosis in patients with NAFLD.[90] However, no evidence is available in older patients with diabetes.

A novel agent for the treatment of NAFLD is the insulin-sensitizer farnesoid X recep-tor ligand obeticholic acid, which is a synthetic variant of the natural bile acid heno-deoxycholic acid.[90] In a multicenter, randomized, placebo-controlled (FLINT) trial involving nearly 300 individuals with noncirrhotic NASH (~16% with established type 2 diabetes), obeticholic acid treatment was associated with resolution of NASH and improvement in fibrosis over 72 weeks of follow-up.[90] However, concerns on long-term safety features (pruritus, increased low-density lipoprotein–cholesterol levels) need to be addressed.[90] In addition, notably, no evidence is available in older patients with diabetes.

Promising agents with anti-inflammatory, antifibrotic, or insulin-sensitizing properties are also being studies in late-phase randomized clinical trials involving patients with NASH.[90]

To date, tailored pharmacotherapy for NAFLD patients with and without type 2 diabetes is a relevant and important clinical challenge. Such aspect seems particularly true for elderly patients who have serious comorbidities and are treated with multiple drugs. For such reasons, the authors believe that the peculiarities of geriatric patients should be always kept in mind by clinicians in the management of NAFLD in these patients. In this regard, a multidisciplinary team involving specialists in hepatology, endocrinology, cardiology, nephrology, and geriatrics is recommended.

SUMMARY

Aging and type 2 diabetes are 2 important economic and social challenges to date.[10] Elderly patients and individuals with type 2 diabetes have a substantial burden of NASH, advanced fibrosis, cirrhosis, and HCC, along with an increased risk of serious extrahepatic complications, including cardiorenal disease.[57-60] For these reasons, the identification and management of NAFLD are clinically relevant to date. Careful consideration of the aspects that characterize elderly individuals (eg, sarcopenia, frailty, dementia, multimorbidity, and polypharmacy) is required.

Appropriate treatment strategies should consider the specific characteristics of the geriatric population and should require a multidisciplinary approach. Nonpharmacologic treatment should be individually tailored considering the physical limitations of most elderly people and the necessity for an adequate caloric supply in most cases.[10] In the same way, the choice for drug therapy should carefully balance in terms of adverse events and pharmacologic interactions.[10] Further epidemiologic and pathophysiologic insights are timely needed in this patient group.

DISCLOSURE

The authors have nothing to disclose.

REFERENCES

1. Younossi Z, Anstee QM, Marietti M, et al. Global burden of NAFLD and NASH: trends, predictions, risk factors and prevention. Nat Rev Gastroenterol Hepatol 2018;15:11–20.

2. Fazel Y, Koenig AB, Sayiner M, et al. Epidemiology and natural history of non-alcoholic fatty liver disease. Metabolism 2016;65:1017–25.

3. Araújo AR, Rosso N, Bedogni G, et al. Global epidemiology of non-alcoholic fatty liver disease/non-alcoholic steatohepatitis: what we need in the future. Liver Int 2018;38(Suppl 1):47–51.

4. Younossi ZM, Koenig AB, Abdelatif D, et al. Global epidemiology of nonalcoholic fatty liver disease–meta-analytic assessment of prevalence, incidence, and outcomes. Hepatology 2016;64:73–84.

5. Targher G, Lonardo A, Byrne CD. Nonalcoholic fatty liver disease and chronic vascular complications of diabetes mellitus. Nat Rev Endocrinol 2018;14:99–114.

6. Younossi ZM, Golabi P, de Avila L, et al. The global epidemiology of NAFLD and NASH in patients with type 2 diabetes: a systematic review and meta-analysis. J Hepatol 2019;71:793–801.

7. Dulai PS, Singh S, Patel J, et al. Increased risk of mortality by fibrosis stage in nonalcoholic fatty liver disease: systematic review and meta-analysis. Hepatology 2017;65:1557–65.

8. Ekstedt M, Hagström H, Nasr P, et al. Fibrosis stage is the strongest predictor for disease-specific mortality in NAFLD after up to 33 years of follow-up. Hepatology 2015;61:1547–54.

9. Vilar-Gomez E, Calzadilla-Bertot L, Wai-Sun Wong V, et al. Fibrosis severity as a determinant of cause-specific mortality in patients with advanced nonalcoholic fatty liver disease: a multi-national cohort study. Gastroenterology 2018;155: 443–57.

10. Bertolotti M, Lonardo A, Mussi C, et al. Nonalcoholic fatty liver disease and aging: epidemiology to management. World J Gastroenterol 2014;20:14185–204.

11. Estes C, Anstee QM, Arias-Loste MT, et al. Modeling NAFLD disease burden in China, France, Germany, Italy, Japan, Spain, United Kingdom, and United States for the period 2016-2030. J Hepatol 2018;69:896–904.

12. Chalasani N, Younossi Z, Lavine JE, et al. The diagnosis and management of nonalcoholic fatty liver disease: practice guidance from the American Association for the Study of Liver Diseases. Hepatology 2018;67:328–57.

13. European Association for the Study of the Liver (EASL); European Association for the Study of Diabetes (EASD); European Association for the Study of Obesity (EASO). EASL-EASD-EASO clinical practice guidelines for the management of non-alcoholic fatty liver disease. J Hepatol 2016;64:1388–402.

14. Kagansky N, Levy S, Keter D, et al. Non-alcoholic fatty liver disease–a common and benign finding in octogenarian patients. Liver Int 2004;24:588–94.

15. Park SH, Jeon WK, Kim SH, et al. Prevalence and risk factors of non-alcoholic fatty liver disease among Korean adults. J Gastroenterol Hepatol 2006;21: 138–43.

16. Karnikowski M, Córdova C, Oliveira RJ, et al. Non-alcoholic fatty liver disease and metabolic syndrome in Brazilian middle-aged and older adults. Sao Paulo Med J 2007;125:333–7.

17. Frith J, Day CP, Henderson E, et al. Non-alcoholic fatty liver disease in older people. Gerontology 2009;55:607–13.

18. Mantovani A, Zoppini G, Targher G, et al. Non-alcoholic fatty liver disease is independently associated with left ventricular hypertrophy in hypertensive type 2 diabetic individuals. J Endocrinol Invest 2012;35:215–8.

19. Koehler EM, Schouten JN, Hansen BE, et al. Prevalence and risk factors of nonalcoholic fatty liver disease in the elderly: results from the Rotterdam study. J Hepatol 2012;57:1305–11.

20. Noureddin M, Yates KP, Vaughn IA, et al, NASH CRN. Clinical and histological determinants of nonalcoholic steatohepatitis and advanced fibrosis in elderly patients. Hepatology 2013;58:1644–54.

21. Lazo M, Hernaez R, Eberhardt MS, et al. Prevalence of nonalcoholic fatty liver disease in the United States: the Third National Health and Nutrition Examination Survey, 1988-1994. Am J Epidemiol 2013;178:38–45.

22. Golabi P, Paik J, Reddy R, et al. Prevalence and long-term outcomes of nonalcoholic fatty liver disease among elderly individuals from the United States. BMC Gastroenterol 2019;19:56.

23. Estes C, Razavi H, Loomba R, et al. Modeling the epidemic of nonalcoholic fatty liver disease demonstrates an exponential increase in burden of disease. Hepatology 2018;67:123–33.

24. Alam S, Fahim SM, Chowdhury MAB, et al. Prevalence and risk factors of non-alcoholic fatty liver disease in Bangladesh. JGH Open 2018;2:39–46.

25. Mantovani A, Byrne CD, Bonora E, et al. Nonalcoholic fatty liver disease and risk of incident type 2 diabetes mellitus: a meta-analysis. Diabetes Care 2018;41: 372–82.

26. Ballestri S, Zona S, Targher G, et al. Nonalcoholic fatty liver disease is associated with an almost twofold increased risk of incident type 2 diabetes and metabolic syndrome. Evidence from a systematic review and meta-analysis. J Gastroenterol Hepatol 2016;31:936–44.

27. Nascimbeni F, Ballestri S, Machado MV, et al. Clinical relevance of liver histopathology and different histological classifications of NASH in adults. Expert Rev Gastroenterol Hepatol 2018;12:351–67.

28. Bazick J, Donithan M, Neuschwander-Tetri BA, et al. Clinical model for NASH and advanced fibrosis in adult patients with diabetes and NAFLD: guidelines for referral in NAFLD. Diabetes Care 2015;38:1347–55.

29. McPherson S, Hardy T, Henderson E, et al. Evidence of NAFLD progression from steatosis to fibrosing-steatohepatitis using paired biopsies: implications for prognosis and clinical management. J Hepatol 2015;62:1148–55.

30. Loomba R, Abraham M, Unalp A, et al, Nonalcoholic Steatohepatitis Clinical Research Network. Association between diabetes, family history of diabetes, and risk of nonalcoholic steatohepatitis and fibrosis. Hepatology 2012;56:943–51.

31. Puchakayala BK, Verma S, Kanwar P, et al. Histopathological differences utilizing the nonalcoholic fatty liver disease activity score criteria in diabetic (type 2 diabetes mellitus) and non-diabetic patients with nonalcoholic fatty liver disease. World J Hepatol 2015;7:2610–8.

32. De Fré CH, De Fré MA, Kwanten WJ, et al. Sarcopenia in patients with non-alcoholic fatty liver disease: is it a clinically significant entity? Obes Rev 2019; 20:353–63.

33. Cruz-Jentoft AJ, Baeyens JP, Bauer JM, et al, European Working Group on Sarcopenia in Older People. Sarcopenia: European consensus on definition and diagnosis: report of the European Working Group on Sarcopenia in older people. Age Ageing 2010;39:412–23.

34. Hong HC, Hwang SY, Choi HY, et al. Relationship between sarcopenia and nonalcoholic fatty liver disease: the Korean Sarcopenic Obesity Study. Hepatology 2014;59:1772–8.

35. Lee YH, Jung KS, Kim SU, et al. Sarcopaenia is associated with NAFLD independently of obesity and insulin resistance: nationwide surveys (KNHANES 2008-2011). J Hepatol 2015;63:486–93.

36. Lee YH, Kim SU, Song K, et al. Sarcopenia is associated with significant liver fibrosis independently of obesity and insulin resistance in nonalcoholic fatty liver disease: nationwide surveys (KNHANES 2008-2011). Hepatology 2016;63: 776–86.

37. Hashimoto Y, Osaka T, Fukuda T, et al. The relationship between hepatic steatosis and skeletal muscle mass index in men with type 2 diabetes. Endocrinol J 2016; 63:877–84.

38. Petta S, Ciminnisi S, Di Marco V, et al. Sarcopenia is associated with severe liver fibrosis in patients with non-alcoholic fatty liver disease. Aliment Pharmacol Ther 2017;45:510–8.

39. Koo BK, Kim D, Joo SK, et al. Sarcopenia is an independent risk factor for non-alcoholic steatohepatitis and significant fibrosis. J Hepatol 2017;66:123–31.

40. Pan X, Han Y, Zou T, et al. Sarcopenia contributes to the progression of nonalco-holic fatty liver disease- related fibrosis: a meta-analysis. Dig Dis 2018;36:427–36.

41. Xia MF, Chen LY, Wu L, et al. The PNPLA3 rs738409 C>G variant influences the association between low skeletal muscle mass and NAFLD: the Shanghai Chang-feng Study. Aliment Pharmacol Ther 2019;50:684–95.

42. Chung GE, Kim MJ, Yim JY, et al. Sarcopenia is significantly associated with pres-ence and severity of nonalcoholic fatty liver disease. J Obes Metab Syndr 2019;28:129–38.

43. Buzzetti E, Pinzani M, Tsochatzis EA. The multiple-hit pathogenesis of non-alcoholic fatty liver disease (NAFLD). Metabolism 2016;65:1038–48.

44. Visser M, Deeg DJ, Lips P, Longitudinal Aging Study Amsterdam. Low vitamin D and high parathyroid hormone levels as determinants of loss of muscle strength and muscle mass (sarcopenia): the Longitudinal Aging Study Amsterdam. J Clin Endocrinol Metab 2003;88:5766–72.

45. Targher G, Scorletti E, Mantovani A, et al. Nonalcoholic fatty liver disease and reduced serum vitamin D(3) levels. Metab Syndr Relat Disord 2013;11:217–28.

46. Biessels GJ, Despa F. Cognitive decline and dementia in diabetes mellitus: mechanisms and clinical implications. Nat Rev Endocrinol 2018;14:591–604.

47. Ghareeb DA, Hafez HS, Hussien HM, et al. Non-alcoholic fatty liver induces insu-lin resistance and metabolic disorders with development of brain damage and dysfunction. Metab Brain Dis 2011;26:253–67.

48. Kim DG, Krenz A, Toussaint LE, et al. Non-alcoholic fatty liver disease induces signs of Alzheimer's disease (AD) in wild-type mice and accelerates pathological signs of AD in an AD model. J Neuroinflammation 2016;13:1.

49. Elliott C, Frith J, Day CP, et al. Functional impairment in alcoholic liver disease and non-alcoholic fatty liver disease is significant and persists over 3 years of follow-up. Dig Dis Sci 2013;58:2383–91.

50. Seo SW, Gottesman RF, Clark JM, et al. Nonalcoholic fatty liver disease is asso-ciated with cognitive function in adults. Neurology 2016;86:1136–42.

51. Celikbilek A, Celikbilek M, Bozkurt G. Cognitive assessment of patients with nonalcoholic fatty liver disease. Eur J Gastroenterol Hepatol 2018;30:944–50.

52. Filipović B, Marković O, Đurić V, et al. Cognitive changes and brain volume reduction in patients with nonalcoholic fatty liver disease. Can J Gastroenterol Hepatol 2018;2018:9638797.

53. Weinstein G, Zelber-Sagi S, Preis SR, et al. Association of nonalcoholic fatty liver disease with lower brain volume in healthy middle-aged adults in the Framingham Study. JAMA Neurol 2018;75:97–104.

54. VanWagner LB, Terry JG, Chow LS, et al. Nonalcoholic fatty liver disease and measures of early brain health in middle-aged adults: the CARDIA study. Obesity (Silver Spring) 2017;25:642–51.

55. Weinstein G, Davis-Plourde K, Himali JJ, et al. Non-alcoholic fatty liver disease, liver fibrosis score and cognitive function in middle-aged adults: the Framingham Study. Liver Int 2019;39:1713–21.

56. Lonardo A, Nascimbeni F, Mantovani A, et al. Hypertension, diabetes, atheroscle-rosis and NASH: cause or consequence? J Hepatol 2018;68:335–52.

57. Anstee QM, Mantovani A, Tilg H, et al. Risk of cardiomyopathy and cardiac ar-rhythmias in patients with nonalcoholic fatty liver disease. Nat Rev Gastroenterol Hepatol 2018;15:425–39.

58. Byrne CD, Targher G. NAFLD: a multisystem disease. J Hepatol 2015;62(1 Suppl):S47–64.

59. Sanyal AJ, Harrison SA, Ratziu V, et al. The natural history of advanced fibrosis due to nonalcoholic steatohepatitis: data from the simtuzumab trials. Hepatology 2019. https://doi.org/10.1002/hep.30664.

60. Loomba R, Adams LA. Editorial: the 20% rule of NASH progression: the natural history of advanced fibrosis and cirrhosis due to NASH. Hepatology 2019. https://doi.org/10.1002/hep.30946.

61. Hui JM, Kench JG, Chitturi S, et al. Long-term outcomes of cirrhosis in nonalcoholic steatohepatitis compared with hepatitis C. Hepatology 2003;38:420–7.

62. Singh S, Allen AM, Wang Z, et al. Fibrosis progression in nonalcoholic fatty liver vs nonalcoholic steatohepatitis: a systematic review and meta-analysis of paired-biopsy studies. Clin Gastroenterol Hepatol 2015;13:643–54.

63. Mantovani A, Targher G. Type 2 diabetes mellitus and risk of hepatocellular carcinoma: spotlight on nonalcoholic fatty liver disease. Ann Transl Med 2017;5:270.

64. Lip GY, Tse HF, Lane DA. Atrial fibrillation. Lancet 2012;379:648–61.

65. Targher G, Mantovani A, Pichiri I, et al. Non-alcoholic fatty liver disease is associated with an increased prevalence of atrial fibrillation in hospitalized patients with type 2 diabetes. Clin Sci (Lond) 2013;125:301–9.

66. Targher G, Valbusa F, Bonapace S, et al. Non-alcoholic fatty liver disease is associated with an increased incidence of atrial fibrillation in patients with type 2 diabetes. PLoS One 2013;8:e57183.

67. Mantovani A, Dauriz M, Sandri D, et al. Association between non-alcoholic fatty liver disease and risk of atrial fibrillation in adult individuals: an updated meta-analysis. Liver Int 2019;39:758–69.

68. Targher G, Valbusa F, Bonapace S, et al. Association of non-alcoholic fatty liver disease with QTc interval in patients with type 2 diabetes. Nutr Metab Cardiovasc Dis 2014;24:663–9.

69. Hung CS, Tseng PH, Tu CH, et al. Nonalcoholic fatty liver disease is associated with QT prolongation in the general population. J Am Heart Assoc 2015;4: e001820.

70. Mantovani A, Rigamonti A, Bonapace S, et al. Nonalcoholic fatty liver disease is associated with ventricular arrhythmias in patients with type 2 diabetes referred for clinically indicated 24-hour Holter monitoring. Diabetes Care 2016;39: 1416–23.

71. Mantovani A, Rigolon R, Pichiri I, et al. Nonalcoholic fatty liver disease is associated with an increased risk of heart block in hospitalized patients with type 2 diabetes mellitus. PLoS One 2017;12:e0185459.

72. Mantovani A, Pernigo M, Bergamini C, et al. Heart valve calcification in patients with type 2 diabetes and nonalcoholic fatty liver disease. Metabolism 2015;64: 879–87.

73. Markus MR, Baumeister SE, Stritzke J, et al. Hepatic steatosis is associated with aortic valve sclerosis in the general population: the Study of Health in Pomerania (SHIP). Arterioscler Thromb Vasc Biol 2013;33:1690–5.

74. Mantovani A, Pernigo M, Bergamini C, et al. Nonalcoholic fatty liver disease is independently associated with early left ventricular diastolic dysfunction in patients with type 2 diabetes. PLoS One 2015;10:e0135329.

75. Mantovani A. Not all NAFLD patients are the same: we need to find a personalized therapeutic approach. Dig Liver Dis 2019;51:176–7.

76. Raschi E, Mazzotti A, Poluzzi E, et al. Pharmacotherapy of type 2 diabetes in patients with chronic liver disease: focus on nonalcoholic fatty liver disease. Expert Opin Pharmacother 2018;19:1903–14.

77. American Diabetes Association. Pharmacologic approaches to glycemic treatment: standards of medical care in diabetes–2018. Diabetes Care 2018;41: S73–85.
78. Cusi K, Orsak B, Bril F, et al. Long-term pioglitazone treatment for patients with nonalcoholic steatohepatitis and prediabetes or type 2 diabetes mellitus: a randomized trial. Ann Intern Med 2016;165:305–15.
79. Musso G, Cassader M, Paschetta E, et al. Thiazolidinediones and advanced liver fibrosis in nonalcoholic steatohepatitis: a meta-analysis. JAMA Intern Med 2017; 177:633–40.
80. Dormandy JA, Charbonnel B, Eckland DJ, et al, PROactive Investigators. Secondary prevention of macrovascular events in patients with type 2 diabetes in the PROactive Study (PROspective pioglitAzone Clinical Trial in macroVascular Events): a randomised controlled trial. Lancet 2005;366:1279–89.
81. Kernan WN, Viscoli CM, Furie KL, et al, IRIS Trial Investigators. Pioglitazone after ischemic stroke or transient ischemic attack. N Engl J Med 2016;374:1321–31.
82. Amstrong MJ, Houlihan DD, Rowe IA, et al. Safety and efficacy of liraglutide in patients with type 2 diabetes and elevated liver enzymes: individual patient data meta-analysis of the LEAD program. Aliment Pharmacol Ther 2013;37: 234–42.
83. Shao N, Kuang HY, Hao M, et al. Benefits of exenatide on obesity and nonalcoholic fatty liver disease with elevated liver enzymes in patients with type 2 diabetes. Diabetes Metab Res Rev 2014;30:521–9.
84. Armstrong MJ, Gaunt P, Aithal GP, Barton D, Hull D, Parker R, Hazlehurst JM, Guo K, LEAN trial team, Abouda G, Aldersley MA, Stocken D, Gough SC, Tomlinson JW, Brown RM, Hübscher SG, Newsome PN. Liraglutide safety and efficacy in patients with non-alcoholic steatohepatitis (LEAN): a multicentre, double-blind, randomised, placebo-controlled phase 2 study. Lancet 2016;387: 679–90.
85. Marso SP, Daniels GH, Brown-Frandsen K, et al, LEADER Steering Committee, LEADER Trial Investigators. Liraglutide and cardiovascular outcomes in type 2 diabetes. N Engl J Med 2016;375:311–22.
86. Kristensen SL, Rørth R, Jhund PS, et al. Cardiovascular, mortality, and kidney outcomes with GLP-1 receptor agonists in patients with type 2 diabetes: a systematic review and meta-analysis of cardiovascular outcome trials. Lancet Diabetes Endocrinol 2019;7:776–85.
87. Cui J, Philo L, Nguyen P, et al. Sitagliptin vs. placebo for non-alcoholic fatty liver disease: a randomized controlled trial. J Hepatol 2016;65:369–76.
88. Hanssen NM, Jandeleit-Dahm KA. Dipeptidyl peptidase-4 inhibitors and cardiovascular and renal disease in type 2 diabetes: what have we learned from the CARMELINA trial? Diab Vasc Dis Res 2019;16:303–9.
89. Katsiki N, Perakakis N, Mantzoros C. Effects of sodium-glucose co-transporter-2 (SGLT2) inhibitors on non-alcoholic fatty liver disease/non-alcoholic steatohepatitis: ex quo et quo vadimus? Metabolism 2019;98:iii–ix.
90. Sumida Y, Yoneda M. Current and future pharmacological therapies for NAFLD/ NASH. J Gastroenterol 2018;53:362–76.

Printed and bound by CPI Group (UK) Ltd, Croydon, CR0 4YY

03/10/2024

01040482-0014